Praise for *The Murmur of Eve*

The Murmur of Everything Moving is a rare love story. Tender, incredibly wise, surprisingly funny, fizzing with youthful desire and impressive courage, this riveting memoir of a twenty-something couple facing mortality far too young is indelible. A story of love as ardent obligation, and of one couple's efforts to defy the odds, this book will change you, for the better.

—**EJ Levy,** author of NYT Editor's Choice novel, *The Cape Doctor,* Lambda-winning *Tasting Life Twice,* and *Love, In Theory*

What I loved most about *The Murmur of Everything Moving* was the way it moved along the same storm systems of high agony and the quiet routine of daily despair—just like the terrible diagnosis it describes. It is moving and tortuous without being cloying or sentimental. The ending is simple and spare and poignant and made my mouth go dry.

—**Lisa Taddeo,** author of NYT best-selling nonfiction book, *Three Women,* and the novels *Animal* and *Ghost Lover.*

THE MURMUR OF
EVERYTHING MOVING

a memoir

MAUREEN STANTON

Columbus State University
PRESS

Library of Congress Control Number: 2024947505

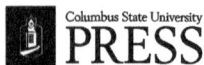

Columbus State University
PRESS

Published by Columbus State University Press

Marketing and distribution by UGA Press

Cover designed by Peter Selgin

Author photo by Heather Perry

Table of Contents

PART I 1
Prologue 3
1. Hitching Post 5
2. What Love Is 15
3. The Steves 25
4. Creature Stealing Up 33
5. Love is Bountiful 39
6. A Tiny Dark Ship 47
7. Paddle 59
8. Thy Known Self 65

PART II 69
9. Flintstones Chewables 71
10. Body Snatchers 81
11. Forget-me-nots 95
12. Zion 103
13. There, There 111
14. Cancer Man 123
15. Motherlode 141
16. Case of the Nosy Neighbors 145
17. Dunleavy Lane 155
18. The Murmur of Everything Moving 167
19. Brompton's Cocktail 181
20. The Price is Right 187
21. Self-deliverance 191
22. Checklist 201
23. Purple Loosestrife 211
24. In the Dawn He Sails Away 217

PART II 225
25. Monochrome 227
26. California 231
27. Driving and Crying 235
28. Jitterbug 241
Coda 249
Acknowledgments 251
About the Author 253

PART I

Prologue

In a home movie of me when I was six, I'm walking down a sidewalk with Frankie S., the boy next door, our movements rapid and jerky in the 8mm film. I'm wearing shorts and a sleeveless shirt so it's probably summer 1966. Frankie has a cowlick, ears that stick out, and tanned skin, which my father calls "dirty" (as if Frankie could scrub off his olive complexion, my father with his pasty Irish skin, pale like waxed paper). Frankie has green eyes, and dimples that give him an impish smile. He's one year younger than me, the same age as my sister, Joanne, who is walking behind us. I have my arm around him possessively, making it clear that Frankie is *mine*.

Frankie is my height, but in my admiring gaze I appear to be looking up at him, my head tilted, smiling adoringly. Through the scratches and blips in the flickering reel, there is no mistaking how smitten I am, which seems amplified by the silence. Each time my family dusts off and watches these home movies, they tease me mercilessly about this scene. *Goo-goo eyes!* They howl with laughter.

When I see that girl goofy with infatuation, I am mortified by my unabashed expression of love. But when I get over the embarrassment, I'm awash in a feeling so familiar that it reminds me of myself, a recognition that cuts through whatever illusions I hold about who I've become (mature, controlled, subtle). My exterior has changed in the decades since I was googly over Frankie, but the heart beating inside is the same.

Some people are fools for love.

Like Steve: Is it foolish to leave a troubled marriage because you *dreamed* one night you were in love with a woman, a sensation so real that when you woke you went in search of her?

Like me: Is it foolish to throw all your belongings into the back of a pick-up truck and move 1,000 miles away with a man you fell in love with in two weeks, and had known for only two months?

Like Steve and me: Is it foolish to give your girlfriend a diamond ring when you are dying? Is it foolish to accept?

For centuries, writers and poets and philosophers have sought to *know* love. The Greeks imposed order on the heart's chaos, a taxonomy: *philia*, brotherly love; *agape*, charitable love—with no return, no questions asked; and *eros*, erotic love. When I met Steve, at 27 he wanted, for the first time in his life, to find love. At 23, full of myself, I thought I knew what love was. In time, we would both learn about love, the hard way.

1. Hitching Post

S teve appeared first as a silhouette, pausing in the threshold of the Hitching Post in Wappingers Falls, New York, where I tended bar in the early 1980s, a post-college stint until I could find a real job. My mother and her boyfriend, Ed, had opened the place a couple years earlier, transforming a burned-out building in to a quaint neighborhood pub, with gingham curtains, a juke box, a six-foot screen for football games, and a thick pine-slab bar with a dozen stools.

Steve stood in the doorway that afternoon, watchful and stealthy in a way that fooled you, as if you suddenly noticed a fox at the edge of the woods who'd been there all along. When you finally saw him, the landscape was altered, contained more than you thought it did.

Tall and lean, broad-shouldered, he wore steel-toed boots and a Carharrt jacket— construction work attire. He strolled up to the bar and ordered a beer. "Is your name Suzie?" he asked.

I blushed, an involuntary response when I met exceptionally handsome men, like Steve with his intense blue eyes, his face almost pretty.

"No, but I have a sister Susan."

"Too bad," he said, smiling.

He left soon after, but returned near midnight, wearing jeans, a yellow jersey the color of his wild curly hair, and a big-collared, bone-white cardigan. He looked like he should be in front of a fireplace with a snifter of brandy, a model in an upscale men's catalog. He looked like a man, not a boy; that's the difference the sweater made. I chatted with him, in between waiting on a handful of customers at that hour, a few solitary men hunched on bar stools, nursing beers, a Hopper-esque tableaux, the neon-orange light from a Budweiser sign blinking in the window.

Steve was an electrician from Michigan who'd traveled to New York for a temporary job arranged by his union. He'd been in New York for a few months by then, late March 1984. He was soft-spoken, his voice low, like purring. I liked his calm, which I took for confidence. My baseline state was anxious, or self-conscious, trying to appear "laid back," which I never was; it was against my nature. I told Steve that I missed the presence of women in my life; the bar's clientele was mostly men, often correctional officers from the two prisons within a mile from the place, who drained scotch and waters after their shifts at 3:00 p.m. and 11:00 p.m., tucking plastic drink stirrers in their shirt pockets like tokens; or at lunch, a rush of steelworkers rebuilding the Newburgh Beacon bridge, who mobbed the joint for a mad half-hour, downing quick beers and burgers, then clearing out like a flock; or after dinner, a few commuters off the train from New York City stopping in for a drink on their way to their suburban homes; and always a smattering of regulars who lived in an apartment complex down the road. The occasional stranger. The occasional woman, most often the girlfriend or wife of some guy.

"I miss my four sisters," I told Steve. "We have silly times." I'm the middle of five girls, close in age. Three of us were in high school and college together. My two brothers are younger.

Steve cocked his head. "Maybe we could have silly times.

I paused, admiring his handsome face, his goofy grin, his two front teeth slightly overlapping, a sensuous mouth, like Marlon Brando.

"Maybe," I said.

He sipped a beer until closing at 3:00 a.m., then watched as I emptied ashtrays and wiped down the bar, lifted chairs onto tables to mop the floor. I appreciated that he didn't offer to help, suggesting I needed it. I had my routine and I was fast and efficient and strong.

When I was done he invited me for a drink.

There are moments in our lives when the wick of desire is lit, when standing on a threshold we glimpse possibility, a larger world that awaits us, and we are forever changed. These glimmers occur unbidden, like the time I was six and my parents threw a cocktail party for the neighbors in our brand-new subdivision, the first adult party I'd seen. I sat on the stairs and spied into the living room, studying the grown-ups until I was caught and sent back to bed.

I remember thinking that adulthood would involve holding short, heavy glasses (not plastic tumblers with built-in straws), swirling the ice cubes in a cocktail, whatever that was. I'd wear flouncy dresses and toss my head back in laughter, blithe and merry. I'd eat only foods I liked, meals of candy and cupcakes, not stew or boiled dinner. And there would be laughing and mysterious games played after children were sent to bed.

When I reached adolescence, my parents divorced and my father moved out of our house, out of my daily life. My heart was broken then, at aged twelve, and the expectation that life could bring sorrow was born, a lesson in loss. I longed to retreat back to the shelter of childhood then, or to be thrust into maturity, to be anywhere but the bardo of adolescence where suddenly I was a stranger to myself.

Even after graduating from college I didn't feel like an adult. I was still waiting for my real life to come around the corner, like an elaborate float in a parade, or a diorama that included all the things adults had: spouses, new cars, homes, important work. Writing figured into the hazy romance of my future, though I had no practical idea of how one became a writer. I longed for a sophisticated life filled with intrigue and excitement, social engagements marked on a calendar, stimulating conversation, love. My image of adult life in my early twenties was scarcely altered from the fantasy I'd imagined as a child.

I was tottering on this verge after college, working as a bartender to save money, to travel, to begin the adventure. I was fueled with hope and ambition and fear as I faced that singular challenge—what to make of one's life—when I met Steve.

Steve and I were the only patrons on the terrace at Cheech's, an after-hours bar. (New York, that licentious state, had no puritanical blue laws forcing bars to close at 1:00 a.m., like in Massachusetts where I grew up.) The cool, pre-dawn air was balmy, weighted, air you could *feel,* air that was itself sensual and erotic. I've always loved that time of night when it seemed that the entire world was asleep, when rules were suspended; you could run a red light, which I did on occasion purely for the pleasure of transgression.

I had the same sensation of breaking rules as I sat outside on Cheech's patio at four in the morning, talking softly with a beautiful curly-haired man, drinking melon balls, a sweet chartreuse concoction: pineapple juice, vodka, and Midori, a honeydew-melon liqueur, like cocktails for children.

"So why did you ask me if my name was Suzie?" I asked Steve, after we settled at our table.

He'd woken up one night from his wife beating on his chest, he explained. He'd been moaning in his sleep, calling *Suzie, Suzie.* Ever since that dream, he'd been asking women—waitresses, clerks, bank tellers—if they were named Suzie, as if the name were a glass slipper.

"You're married," I said, annoyed. "Where's your ring?"

"I don't wear it anymore since my buddy lost his finger." A "hot wire" had shocked his friend at work one day, and the wedding ring had conducted the electricity, super-heating the metal. The story was gruesome, but a reasonable explanation for why he'd left his ring off.

"Besides, we're separated," he said.

I asked him how long he'd been married, as I stirred my drink into a miniature whirlpool.

"Eight years," he said.

Another surprise. Steve sipped his melon ball through the tiny cocktail straw as if he were new at it, just learning. He was, I'd learn, innocent for his age, twenty-seven: he'd never skied down a mountain, never flown in a plane, had made love to just one woman, his wife, who'd been a high school girlfriend.

"I hate my wife," he said casually, as if stating the color of his house, a fact rather than an emotion, a condition to which he'd become inured.

Hate is a strong word, I wanted to say. My mother had banished the word from my vocabulary when I was a girl, insisting it was sinful to hate anyone, threatening to wash my mouth with soap. I found something oddly admirable in Steve's reclamation of this powerful word, his willingness to admit strong—even unbecoming—feelings. He's honest, I thought. Or perhaps just reckless. But I was appalled by his situation. "You've been living with a woman you hate for *eight* years?" I said. "That's sad. You must have loved her at some point."

He'd met Deborah in his senior year of high school at his job in a shoe store. "She came in all the time with her mother. She just kept coming by. Finally I went out with her."

I understood Steve's story because that's how I'd ended up with David, the man I lived with for three years in college, with whom I'd broken up two months earlier. I'd met David in my sophomore year, in a packed dive bar one night, the place everyone went for last call. I'd asked him for a match to light my cigarette; he was the person standing nearest to me. We chatted, and after the bar closed, I saw him walking home on that cold March night, so I offered him a ride. At his apartment, he asked me if I wanted to hear a song he'd written. *Just one song.* I agreed. I stayed the night, one of those regretful drunken youthful decisions (not a decision really, more like curiosity, or yearning for experience). When I left the next day, I had no desire to see David again, but he kept phoning. I asked my roommate to screen his calls, but he got through once because I had a friend from my hometown named David. My roommate got confused.

Musician David convinced me to meet him just one more time so he could thank me for the ride. He reminded me that we'd slept together, that we should meet anyway just to see each other after that intimacy.

As it turned out, David was older, worldly, more interesting than the college boys in my dorm. He was kind, a gifted self-taught musician. I ended up with David by relenting to a steady beat of suggestion, and over time I grew to like, then love him.

Steve had broken up with Deborah after a couple months, then he graduated high school and hit the road. "I went to Colorado," he said. "The spruce trees, the mountains. I loved it." He planned on living there, but one day when he called home to Michigan his father told him that his ex-girlfriend, at 17, was pregnant.

"I didn't know what to do," he said. "Everyone told me I should come home and marry her, that that was the right thing to do."

We were quiet for a moment at our table at Cheech's. Then I asked, "Why did you stay for eight years if you didn't love her?"

"If you marry someone, you're supposed to be committed for life," he said.

Old fashioned, I thought. I respected that he'd taken his vows seriously. Still, I thought his loveless life seemed tragic.

"How can you live without love?" I said, fishing for an ice chip in my drink.

"I don't know what love is," he said, his voice subdued, confessional, as if he were admitting illiteracy.

"*Love,*" I said. "You know, when your heart goes pitter patter. When you get that butterfly feeling in your stomach." That was my definition then, love as an anxiety attack.

He looked at me coolly. "Like I have right now?"

I glanced away, blushing. "Oh, you do not."

We sat in Steve's truck in the parking lot of Cheech's and talked. His second child, a son, was planned; he and Deborah thought another child might help their struggling marriage. His third child, like his first, was an accident. Steve might have stayed in his marriage longer, from inertia, if not for that dream, that haunting beautiful dream. He said he'd never had that feeling before, the feeling he had in his dream of Suzie: passion, or maybe that was love. "That's when I decided to leave," he said. It seemed preposterous that he'd altered the course of his life because of a dream, but I understood his yearning, his simple human bid for a life infused with love.

He told me about his kids, Sarah, Nate, and Lisa, the youngest, just two years old, about her premature birth and near death. Though innocent of the world in some ways, Steve was mature in others. He'd witnessed birth, fathered three children, supported a family, though he confessed to terrible fights with Deborah, screaming fights that upset the kids. He told me about a recent trip home, a morning when he'd taken Nate, his four-year-old, for a boat ride in the kettle-hole pond in their backyard. Steve rowed while Nate dragged his fingers in the water trying to catch duck feathers floating on the surface. Steve had asked Nate, "Do you want me to leave?"

I was taken aback. Why would he ask a four-year-old such a portentous question? I didn't know Nate yet, didn't know he was the bellwether child, the sensitive one. Steve told me that Nate was silent, but in the middle of that murky pond in their backyard, surrounded by huge willows weeping their leaves onto the shore, Nate nodded.

Cheech's parking lot was empty—even the bartender was gone. Steve started his truck and we cruised aimlessly along the hilly country roads that dissect the Hudson River valley. We stopped at an all-night market for coffee, my first cup ever—creamy and sweet with three sugars— and I felt like I was on the brink of something addicting, something dangerous but delicious. Down the road, Steve pulled onto the grounds of Tioronda, an ornate Civil-war era, Gothic mansion, closed then but once a private sanitarium for the wealthy—Zelda Fitzgerald, Rosemary Kennedy, Truman Capote, and Marilyn Monroe were said to have spent time there.

We sat quietly in the driveway. Outside, the dawn mist made everything dreamy. A deer grazing on the grounds eyed us but didn't leap away, as if drugged by the watery smoke. The doe ambled off on legs swallowed by fog, its body floating, moving the way I felt. Vapor fumed from the surface of the Hudson and lingered in the air like a presence.

"I want you to meet Arnie and Red," Steve said, abruptly, starting the engine. "That's crazy," I said. "It's nearly 5:00 a.m." But he wasn't worried. "They won't mind," he said. "They love me." He steered the truck onto Route 9D, and ten minutes later we were knocking on an apartment door. A groggy but surprisingly pleasant rumpled-haired Arnie invited us inside. Arnie's wife, Red, emerged from the bedroom, pulling on her robe. She hugged Steve.

"I found Suzie!" Steve said.

Arnie and Red looked me over, wondering probably why I'd been chosen, anointed almost, by Steve. I didn't know yet about the other women he'd been dating while working in New York, a school teacher, an office worker. How many other Suzies had be brought before his friends?

We chatted with Arnie in their living room while Red fried eggs and then morning arrived suddenly, hot sun beaming in the bay window. Steve rested his head on my shoulder, which was the first time he touched me ever.

After breakfast, Steve dropped me off in the parking lot of the Hitching Post, where I'd left my car. "Well, goodbye," I said, sliding one leg out the truck door.

"Can I have a kiss?" he said, as if he were asking for a stick of gum.

I'd been kissing boys since seventh grade, then men. None of them had ever asked, only taken kisses, often in oafish drunken lunges (the junior high boys more graceful than some in college). I studied Steve for a moment, his fine straight nose, high broad forehead, that beguiling grin.

"Okay," I said. We kissed lightly on the lips.

"Can I have another?" he asked.

That kiss, that sweet tender touch, tilted the trajectory of my life.

2. What Love Is

When I was six, my babysitter Ann and her boyfriend, Ned, took me and my then five siblings swimming at Aho Grove across town. We were Ann and Ned's pretend children; they were practicing being adults, playing wife and husband. We walked down a narrow path that opened up to a small beach, a big lake. I was in heaven. I loved to swim. I immediately jumped in the warm brownish-green water. The bottom of the pond was not squishy, which I hated, but sandy. I waded far out, up to my neck, then bobbed up and down, imagining myself a spring from inside a ball point pen. I could hold my breath underwater for a long time—"Watch me!" I shouted—but Ann was busy with her boyfriend. It was plain they were in love, holding hands and kissing.

I popped out of the water again, but this time I accidentally stepped off the shelf of sand at the bottom and then I was floating down like a curled brown leaf in autumn, sinking slowly. There was no ground beneath me. The air was thick and yellowish, but it wasn't air, it was water. I could see the sun shimmering above my head, blurry and wobbly. I couldn't reach it, but it was so quiet and I was dreamy and sleepy, then everything went black.

Suddenly I felt cold air. Someone had grabbed me by the back of my one piece bathing suit and had me in his strong arms. It was Ned, Ann's boyfriend. Then I was choking and coughing and crying, and Ann swaddled me in a huge towel as if she were rolling me in a rug. Ned picked me up and carried me in his arms, and he and Ann walked up the path to a small cottage. My siblings, draped in towel-capes, waddled behind like goslings.

Ann was singing her favorite song, my mother's, too, by Dean Martin, whom they adored. *Everybody / loves somebody / sometime.* Ann had a beautiful smoky voice. Ned sang too, and I could feel the warm words vibrate in his chest, could see the tiny crabapple in his throat darting, he was holding me that tight, and I felt happy and safe. *I* was the one Ned was singing to, *I* was the *somebody* whom everybody loved.

He set me on a bed in the cottage and I slept deeply. When I woke up, it was dark and I was hazy. For a long time after, I associated loving somebody with that feeling of drowning.

I don't know what love is. I mulled Steve's words from that night in Cheech's. I felt sorry for him, that he'd never known love. I liked that he candidly admitted his inexperience, unconcerned that I might find him wanting romantically.

My own romantic education was empirical and early, however flawed, starting with Dennis T. in eighth grade. In a throe of desire one Saturday afternoon I was compelled to scrawl "Maureen + Dennis, TLA" (True Love Always) fifty times on the walls of the ladies room of Friendly's restaurant. My love seemed as indelible as the ink: love writ large in green magic marker. Both faded eventually, my love and its declaration, though not before I'd wept for three days in the cafeteria after Dennis dumped me for Lisa H., the new girl with waist-length blonde hair. I could not fathom that for some, love was so ephemeral, so *replaceable*, as I watched Dennis with Lisa at the couple's table in the lunchroom, in the seat I had so recently occupied.

Then there was Nicky in high school, an ethereal angel of a boy with silky blonde hair to his shoulders, and smooth flawless skin. At sixteen, like every disenfranchised teenager in Massachusetts it seemed, we dreamed of running away to California, that sunny golden state. Nicky and I became pre-engaged one Christmas when he gave me a diamond-chip ring with tiny heart cut-outs in the gold band. We set a sensible date, two years after high school graduation. I wrote it on my bedroom wall, but we didn't last another six months.

David, my boyfriend in college, was the man who'd kindled our relationship with a match to my cigarette, a flint that sparked our three-years together. David was ten years older than me, a songwriter with a powerful baritone voice that belied his small stature. He'd grown up in Puerto Rico, but left home at fifteen to escape beatings by his father. He'd wandered homeless on the streets of Argentina and Chile, joined the Children of God, a missionary group (cult, more accurately), and had traveled extensively in South America.

By the time I met David he was a member of the Sufi order, following the teachings of Hazrat Inayat Khan. (Daoud was his Sufi name, but I never called him that.) He gave me a book of poems by Rumi, and memoir by Reshad Feild, *The Last Barrier*, about Feild's spiritual journey and conversion to Sufism. The book was compelling, with stories of mystical sects and fantastic coincidences (that were not coincidences at all), whirling dervishes, and the recurring image of a beautiful woman Feild saw periodically in his "faith trip," who was constantly trying to untangle a length of blue yarn.

David played music in coffee houses around town, meditated and prayed, at least when he wasn't on a drinking binge. I apprenticed to David in love and sex and eastern philosophy for three years, until I realized he was an alcoholic. It took me a while to realize I couldn't save David, especially as he wasn't trying to save himself.

After I left David, I vowed to remain single for two years, to focus on writing and creative projects with my artist sister, Sally. But in spite of my oath, I went on a several dates before I met Steve. There was Kurt, a nuclear engineer who piloted his own plane and promised to give me flying lessons. He looked like Clark Kent, with black-framed glasses, small blue eyes, thin lips, a sharp nose. He drank Spaten, an imported

German lager, so I nicknamed him Uberman. When he was drunk, sitting for hours on a barstool at the Hitching Post, Kurt tried to cajole me into a *ménage à trois* with he and his ex-wife, which I'd politely decline. I agreed to date him because he was so insistent, but also he was smart and we sometimes had interesting conversations. Kurt showed up with a single red rose and a box of chocolates, and we dined at a fancy restaurant. He politely kissed my cheek at the end of the night. He was thoughtful and sweet, but the date was boring. I was never a flowers-and-candy kind of girl.

Another man invited me to sail to the Bahamas; he was first-mate to a captain named Cliff, who chartered the sloop Clearwater, in the Hudson, and knew folk singer, Pete Seeger. I liked the sailor, but we'd be trapped on a boat for weeks, along with Cliff and his girlfriend. Clearly I was meant to be his sea-faring paramour. What if I said no? Would he toss me overboard, or leave me stranded at some remote port?

There was Andy, an air traffic controller whose sense of humor matched mine. On our dinner date he drank heavily, and instead of dropping me off at my car at the Hitching Post, as I'd asked, he whizzed past and onto his apartment complex. In the parking lot he tried to strong-arm me (literally) into coming inside, pressed himself against me until I pushed him away angrily. I said I'd walk home, so he finally gave me a ride. When he next came into the bar he acted annoyed, as if I'd cheated him of something.

There was James, who had a master's degree in sociology, but worked as a waiter at a four–star restaurant. James took me to a country inn for lunch. Strolling through the restaurant's gardens after eating, he took my hand, which felt too intimate. After a minute, I told him I wasn't comfortable holding hands. I felt miserly—it was just a hand—but also relieved when I freed my palm from his sweaty grip.

There was the handsome 30-year-old salt-and-pepper-haired stock broker, with the plain name of Peter Jones, who'd stop by for a drink between the train station in Beacon and his home, where his wife waited. He began coming in later on some nights, stayed till closing, chatted me up as I cleaned. Once he followed me in the men's room as I mopped, and invited me to meet him at a hotel. It was almost a dare. We made a plan, but it snowed that night and we cancelled, which was a relief. It prevented his adultery (at least with me), and gave me time to rethink that ill-conceived tryst, to recognize my naiveté and selfishness.

There were others. I didn't really want to be in a relationship, but the attention was heady—even under the circumstances; I knew that the bartender always gets asked out. At the Hitching Post, men were everywhere and interested. But I could sense in those men some edge of desperation, some tinge of need that was off-putting.

Then there was Steve, so cool, so calm, with a palpable presence when he walked into the room, as if he'd molecularly changed the air around him, electrically charged it—tall and lean, graceful and quiet, beautiful in a way that I am sometimes astonished humans can be, but unselfconscious. He was unpretentious and playful, masculine and boyish at the same time.

After that night at Cheech's, for our first date Steve invited me to play Frisbee, an offer that was perfectly suited to me. I'd taken a Frisbee class in college—a one-credit gym class—and learned ten ways of throwing the Frisbee, and freestyle tricks. I owned a professional-weight disc. I was *good* at Frisbee. I'd had a Frisbee injury—a fractured ulna from vying to catch the disc against a large man who accidentally bumped me to the pavement. I landed on my elbow. My right arm in a sling, I learned the ten tosses with my left hand and earned an A in the class. When Steve asked me on a date to play Frisbee, of course I said yes. No boring dinner for us. Steve didn't try to impress me (that impressed me).

After that date, Steve and I spent all our free time together. We drove around in his dragonfly-green Jeep pickup truck. One day when I got into the truck, he said, "You're so far away. Why don't you slide on over?" I never pictured myself as the sort of woman who sat glued to her boyfriend in the front seat of a pick-up truck; I'd never had a boyfriend with a pickup truck. But when Steve invited me over, suddenly that gulf of vinyl between us seemed impossibly wide. I scooched over.

Steve and I went everywhere in that truck and everywhere we went felt like an adventure. Steve was on his own for the first time since his foreshortened trip to Colorado when he was eighteen, so he wanted to live fully, making up for lost time, his unspent youth. He was like a wide-eyed kid, absorbing it all. We went skiing one weekend, the first time for Steve. He slid off the chairlift then glided backwards down the hill until he fell, laughing.

We drove winding one-lane roads listening to my cassettes, Mozart and Beethoven (Steve had never paid attention to classical music), or British new wave (new to him, also). We slow-danced in a deserted bar in some small town. The only other patrons, an older couple, watched us appreciatively, recalling perhaps their own courting. We toured Brotherhood Winery in Washingtonville, New York, the oldest winery in the country, and got tipsy on medicine-cup-sized pours, brought home bottles of sweet May wine. We grilled-out in deserted state parks in the still chilly spring weather, spent a day at Bear Mountain park hiking, then watching the monkeys in the zoo. During Steve's break on the night shift, I'd bring dinner to the construction site. We'd spread a blanket on a swath of grass in the parking lot and picnicked beneath the greenish glare of sodium lights.

After my shifts at the Hitching post at three a.m., I'd drive to Steve's apartment in the end-unit of a small motel, tiptoe past Five Noses, the snoring desk clerk so named for his bulbous, ruddy nose, and crawl into bed with Steve, redolent as I was of cigarettes and stale beer. In the morning, I'd open my eyes to Steve's face inches from mine, his head resting in the palm of his hand, studying me like I was sculpture. I'd pull close to his warm body, inhaling his scent, which was salty and sour, pungent, like stepping on skunk cabbage in the woods.

Steve lured me out of my cave of sleep with caresses. It was a drug I couldn't get enough of, the affection narcotic. David had not been affectionate. If I asked for a kiss, he'd sigh and sometimes indulge me, but he thought my need was childish. I never knew what it was like to be adored, to be that sole center of someone's attention, to be doted on—until I met Steve. He complimented me, said I was beautiful, said I was smart, said he was lucky.

We kissed languidly, as if we were slowly devouring each other.

"That kiss was like taking a bite out of a peach," I said once.

"You are a peach," he replied.

After we made love one morning, Steve hopped out of bed. "I'll cook you breakfast," he said.

"You would do that?"

He nodded. "I'm inspiring you to fall in love with me."

I was inspired.

I've fallen in love in two ways, and maybe that's true for most people— in a hurry and over time. In the slow way, typically I'd had little interest in the person (even an active disinterest, as with David), but in those circumstances, as I came to know the person incrementally, I was surprised by a gathering attraction that built into love. The sudden way was surprising for its overpowering urgency: the person entered my life like a bright meteor flaming across the sky, eclipsing everything else. A white-hot love. These "passionate" loves seemed *outside* of myself: ordained. I had no choice. Kismet: like we'd started something in a previous life that needed to be finished. Steve was that kind of love.

In Steve's quest to find "Suzie," the lover in his dream, he'd dated other women since he'd arrived in New York months earlier. He'd been on a mission, searching for love like a Holy Grail, but I was his last stop: I was *her*. The glass slipper fit; we both knew it.

Time seemed to move quickly. Steve gave me a card on Easter Sunday, just three weeks after we met, a silly cartoon man in a bunny suit. The caption: *My mother told me to watch out for girls like you.* Inside: *I have, and they're pretty hard to find.* Inside he'd written a note: "You make me very happy." I was intrigued that he bestowed me with the power to affect his disposition. I could make him *very happy.* This became my mission: to make Steve ecstatic, to introduce him to hedonism, to all that existed beyond the confines of his sad, failing marriage. At twenty-three, I believed that I'd mastered love, as if the subject had come easily to me the way Spanish had in junior high. I was excited about the possibility that I might mentor Steve, induct him into the cult of Eros.

We started with the basics. Sex, Steve confessed, had been a perfunctory act in a loveless marriage, and so I became his guide, mapping my body, naming places, like the *Reader's Digest* articles I loved reading as a girl: "I am Jane's Breast." We took baths together, soaking until our fingers pruned, making love in the tub, creating a series of small tsunamis that spilled onto the tile floor.

In bed one morning Steve traced his fingertip along the fine crow's feet etched around my eyes already. "I think I'm falling in love with you," he said.

"Me too." I sighed.

"You're falling in love with you, too?"

I laughed, but it was true. When someone tells you he loves you, when he exclaims your beauty, the words are transformative. Suddenly, you *are* lovable. Love is reflective: Steve and I were falling in love with ourselves falling in love with each other.

First we were falling; then we fell. By that afternoon, Steve was unequivocal. "I love you," he said. No more *thinking* about it.

"I love you more," I said, upping the ante as if in a card game.

"I love you to the tenth power," he said, compounding, multiplying. As our hearts expanded, our focus narrowed. Nothing existed outside the frame we inhabited. There was us, and there was the rest of the world, dim and blurry in the periphery. We were mutually obsessed, in a shared solipsism. The state of New York was, for us, a *state* of love, like a duty-free zone in the airport, where a conventional logic or order didn't apply. A zone of immunity, far from Michigan where Steve had his past, his unhappy marriage; removed from Boston where my family was, which represented for me settling into a responsible job, measuring up to others' expectations.

Seeking escape from the world, we found refuge in each other. Self-exiled, we spent hours in desolate places, like a dilapidated mansion in Newburgh that overlooked the Hudson, a relic from the heyday of passenger trains when wealthy Manhattanites summered upriver. We climbed into the cracked cement swimming pool, where weeds poked through the fissures, spent hours wandering through the three-story Italianate, peeling curls of mildewed wallpaper, examining artifacts—a shoe, a pot, a plate. We wondered what had caused such a charmed life to come to ruins. The wreck felt romantic to us, perhaps simply because *we* were in it.

Or maybe the dilapidated manor evoked in us a sense of nostalgia. From its beginning, our affair was imbued with a sense of finality, its ending already scripted, almost visible like a distant landscape across a sea. I'd been saving for a backpacking trip across Europe. Steve had to return to Michigan at some point to finalize his divorce. We grieved the end of our relationship even as it was still unfolding. Whenever Steve stopped by the Hitching Post during my shift, he'd drop quarters into the juke box and queue the same song a half-dozen times, *Miss Me Blind* by Boy George, anticipating already how we'd long for each other in the future, nostalgic for a past that wasn't all present yet.

Perhaps because of the uncertainty of an actual future together, we created a fantasy. Each night, just before falling asleep we added chapters to our novel life. We'd live on a secluded patch of land with his kids and one of our own. We never assigned a name to the place—Colorado or Michigan or Massachusetts—and in my mind, the terrain shifted: an island, a sunny meadow, mountains. We'd build our own house, a huge Swiss-family-Robinson tree hut, I envisioned, but Steve saw an earth-berm home, an idea that fascinated him. He loved reading *Mother Earth News*, with its blueprints for windmills and irrigation systems and composting bins. We'd have solar power, live off the grid. We'd fish and hunt, grow vegetables and fruits, harvest grapes for wine, keep bees and collect honey. Steve and I never spoke of bad weather, failed crops, boredom, hours upon hours of labor. We didn't foresee trouble of any kind in our imaginary paradise, not even a bee sting.

Steve, for me, was a haven, his body a sheltering landscape. I adored Steve's muscular form—bulging biceps and triceps from punching a bag for hours every night back in Michigan, years of sparring with dead weight, and from pulling wire on his jobs electrifying industrial buildings. I loved his lanky frame, his long shapely legs, narrow waist, flared deltoids. I never appreciated muscles until I met Steve. With Steve, I felt safe and secure. Once, when a movie theater became insufferably hot and the projectionist failed to respond to the audience's complaints, Steve casually walked up the aisle, picked the lock on the thermostat and lowered the temperature. I liked that he took matters into his own hands.

I liked that he'd dug an entire basement by hand, one shovel-load at a time (he'd shown me before and after pictures of the small, run-down house he'd refurbished and then rented out). I liked that his job as an electrician was dangerous, like flying a kite strung to a key during a lightning storm. He had survival skills, an intuition for engineering, and manual dexterity. Steve was the man with whom I'd want to be marooned, and that was what we envisioned for ourselves on our private homestead. Alone but together. Independent. Self-sufficient. Fortified by love, if the world around us collapsed, we'd survive.

3. The Steves

In mid-May 1984, about eight weeks after I met Steve, I quit my job at the Hitching Post and booked a flight to Europe. Europe was a dream, a goal recorded in my high school year book. My best friend Kathy wrote on the senior class photo she gave me, *see you in Europe.* Now, a year after graduating college, a year of saving nickels and dimes and quarters, my fortune measured in tips that I recorded in a notebook each night after my shift, even at 4:00 a.m., the wages of slinging beer and mixing scotch and sodas—now I could afford my dream. I never said it aloud, but after I'd met Steve and fallen for him so quickly, I half-wished I wasn't going to Europe. But I had a duty to myself, to this long-planned trip.

Before I left, Steve and I traveled for a weekend to Cape Cod where Steve dipped his toe in the Atlantic, the first time he'd seen the ocean. We watched a pod of minke whales feeding offshore in the quiet waters near Provincetown, where the Cape Cod landscape curls into a beckoning finger. We made love under blankets on the deserted Nauset Beach, the open ocean side of the Cape with pounding surf; we were the only souls there in the off season. Then we parted in the driveway of my childhood home where Steve dropped me off before heading back to New York, to finish his job for a few more weeks, and eventually to return to Michigan.

I gave Steve a t-shirt with a decal of lips pressed on the inside of the back collar—a kiss—and a curl of my hair in a matchbox. I took from him an unlaundered shirt suffused with his sour-sweet scent. The bulky shirt burdened my overstuffed backpack, but it evoked Steve; I couldn't discard it. My original plan had been to travel as long as my money lasted, possibly a year—I'd saved $8,000 from sixty-hour work-weeks. I thought maybe I'd find a job in Europe, though I scarcely wanted that anymore.

My sister, Sue, and my high school friend, Kathy, and I traveled together for three weeks, and then I was alone. Coincidentally, Sue and Kathy and I were all dating men named Steve, all of whom were 6'1", all blond and blue-eyed, as if we'd purchased them at the boyfriend store, in the Steve aisle. As we traveled beneath the weight of our backpacks, there was a good deal of conversation about *Steve*.

On our blitz through five countries, I spent my hard-earned savings lavishly, possibly hoping it would be depleted more quickly so I'd have an excuse to return to the states and see Steve. I called him from Italy after an hour-long wait at the public phones, waking him at 3:00 a.m., and then from a hotel in Innsbruck, while the desk clerk frantically waved at me outside the glass-enclosed booth as I ignored the minutes ticking by, accruing enormous surcharges, nearly $100 for ten minutes.

In early June Steve left New York for Michigan; I couldn't call him at his house where he and his wife were working out their divorce. Instead, I wrote him letters every day, addressed to his sister's house, and he wrote back, a stack of envelopes that awaited me at my mother's house. We sent our missives of love and longing into the world, our ephemera traveling slowly, as if by carrier pigeon winging across a sea, neither of us quite receiving the letters until their urgent sentiments were past.

After Sue left first, and days later Kathy flew home from Amsterdam, I wandered alone for a couple weeks. We'd had seventeen consecutive days of rain, so I impulsively boarded a train bound for Spain, backtracking south, heliotropically aiming for sun. In Barcelona, I met Siobhan, an Australian woman also in her early twenties, who'd been backpacking for nine months. Over a pitcher of sangria, she cried about missing her family and friends, but she was intent on completing her year-long journey. Siobhan was me, only braver, more determined; she would continue south to Alicante, and then to Singapore and Malaysia before returning home. I walked her to the youth hostel just before they locked the doors at the midnight curfew. On my way back to my hotel a mile or so away, the streetlights blinked out, an energy-saving measure I guessed, but I became frightened in the dark streets of this foreign city, tipsy from wine, an obvious American tourist: alone, an easy target.

I'd already been talked out of $20 by a respectable-looking, middle-aged Australian man, who'd convinced me he'd been pickpocketed and needed money to get by until the embassy opened on Monday. If he truly needed help, I didn't want to deny him aid, to be unkind to a stranger in need. But I was wary. "If you are scamming me, I will lose my faith in humanity and it will be your fault," I told him. I was naïve enough to think that he would not play fast and loose with a young woman's belief in the goodness of her fellow human. I see now that my warning to him was also a hint to myself, but I ignored my instinct in favor of charity. "Trust me," he said. As I handed him the money, a micro-expression on his face—a twitch in his cheek—revealed instantly, wordlessly his con. He'd taken my twenty bucks, but I decided I wouldn't let him take my faith in people after all.

After dropping off Siobhan that night, after the street lights winked out, I ran. Nobody was chasing me, but I gave myself a head start anyway, sprinting to my cheap hotel, believing I could outrun any trouble. Steve had told me a story about a time he'd gone jogging when he first arrived in New York. He'd gotten lost running in Newburgh, a smallish run-down city on the Hudson River. After a while, he found himself in a sketchy part of town. He hadn't brought any money to call a cab so he just kept running and running as night fell. Eventually, he recognized a building and found his way back to his hotel. When he took his sneakers off his feet were bleeding.

In those three weeks traveling alone I had moments of pure bliss: eating the sweetest sun-warmed strawberries on the beach in Barcelona; traveling by train south along the Costa Brava, flanked by the Pyrenees to the west, the Catalonian hillside splotched with brilliant red poppies, the blue-black waters of the Mediterranean to the east. I spent hours in the Picasso museum surrounded by his mad art, and drank beer at cafés on Las Ramblas in Barcelona, watching the stream of people, the tourists (like me), and handsome young street artists chalking replicas of masterpieces on the sidewalk.

But I also felt lonely and inept, and acted carelessly or did not *take* care. I fell asleep on the beach and was burned so badly I couldn't leave my hotel room for two days. One afternoon, I sat on a rock watching the surf smash into the breakers, feeling the spray on my face. An old man stopped and scolded me. *Peligrosa!* he said. Dangerous. One rogue wave and I'd be rinsed from my perch, lost in the swirling sea foam. An old woman in the hills outside the city where I'd wandered one day tsked at me. *Tu vestida!* She shook her head at my shorts and a tank top.

On my way north at the train station in Narbonne, France across the border from Spain, I waited on the patio for my train. Writing in my journal, I looked up to find myself surrounded by taunting menacing pre-adolescent boys, who poked at me like I was a stray dog. Inside, a waiter took my drink order, only he wasn't a waiter, just a man in a disheveled suit coat (I noticed finally), who brought me tea and said he was a poet. Luckily he was, and later he ran home and brought me a copy of his chapbook.

In London, I met another young woman traveling alone, so we shared a room for two nights, Beverly, from Ohio. She moaned in her sleep and the next day when I asked her about it, she said she'd had her recurring dream of being on a ship, of being raped. She said one night over dinner, "I've never felt beautiful," which made me inordinately sad.

Her father had turned taciturn in his last years, she told me; she'd only understood after his death that a cancer had been eating away his guts; he'd never told his family.

A young Indian man, a waiter in a restaurant where I dined, offered to squire me around a castle in Arundel on England's south shore. After the tour, he asked me to marry him. When I politely said no, he tried to persuade me (as if he could), and then turned angry and stomped off. I was glad to be relieved of him, but I felt bad because someone thought I was that stupid, or that in need of love or a husband that I'd say yes to *any* proposal, that all it would take to snare me (and a green card) was a quick spin around a local tourist spot. Did I look so lonely? Or was it just because I was alone?

I missed Steve. Each night before I fell asleep I'd unreel the filmstrip in my mind of our first moments together, our giddy days of falling in love, our silly times over the two months we'd had. I clutched at memory, etching him in my consciousness, memorizing him, perhaps because I could sense he was fading already. Every moment of my trip was freighted by a sense of expectancy, biding time.

On my last day of solo travel, before I was to meet my father in Ireland for a week, I hung around Covent Garden in London watching street performers. Under a tent bustling with artisans and flea market vendors, I saw a line of women in front of a booth waiting to have their palms read. I half-believed in prophecy, introduced to divination as a girl through my mother's nightstand stash of pocket-editions on palm reading, astrology, and hand-writing analysis. I remember one compelling book titled, *Face Reading: The Chinese Art of Physiognomy*, its pages filled with photos of damning crooked noses and worrisome weak chins, the "hanging needle," a single straight crease between the eyes, a portent of trouble. Most disturbing was a feature that foretold death by tragic circumstances: "three white-sided eyes"—irises surrounded on both sides and the bottom by the sclera, illustrated by photos of JFK and Martin Luther King. Since I had no plans beyond the trip, no idea how to follow my dream of writing or how to fashion a life, unsure if Steve would still love me, if I'd even see him again, I took a place in the queue.

The palm reader was a tiny octogenarian man, Chinese, balding, wearing a cardigan and bedroom slippers. I remained silent as he took my chin in his hand and positioned my face squarely in front of him, like a parent wiping a smudge from my cheek. "Very good face," he said. He held both of my palms in his warm, soft hands, then traced his index finger along the map of lines. "You like to talk. You are witty, but have sharp tongue." Pressing his thumbs into the flesh of my palms, he said, "Trouble and hard times in family at fifteen. Better later. When trouble comes, you get tired and go to bed." I took this to mean the spells of melancholy that sometimes beset me, which started in my teen years after my parents divorced.

The palm reader was uncannily accurate about my personality traits and history, so it was easy to believe him when he spoke of my future. "You will have a house and property. At twenty-five, you'll have a lover," he said, "twenty-seven another lover, thirty another lover," as if he could see their faces in my palms.

"You are in love now," he said.

I smiled.

"It won't last," he said.

I felt sick to my stomach. "But I really love this man."

He consulted my palms. "Maybe six months, maybe a year. No more."

The palm reader predicted I'd have two children, a boy and a girl, that I'd be successful in my own business.

I asked him just one question – would I be a writer?

He looked into my palms. "Hobby only. No money," he said and released my hands. I paid him and rushed out of the curtained booth, pressing back hot tears until I found solitude on the granite stairs of a church, and then I wept. I didn't want to believe that the two things I most wanted—to be a writer, and to be with Steve—he predicted I would not have.

"Failure or success in life is allotted to us by the stars," E. M. Forster wrote, "but we retain the power of wriggling, of fighting with or against our fate." On those stone steps in England in 1984, I wrote the palm reader's predictions in my journal, determined to track my future against them, to prove them wrong, to wriggle against fate.

4. Creature Stealing Up

Eros once again limb-loosener whirls me
sweetbitter, impossible to fight off,
creature stealing up
Sappho

Sweetbitter, Sappho wrote, as if what is dulcet inevitably turns sour. Or perhaps love is bittersweet because its sublime pleasure is tinged by fear of its inevitable loss. My mother told me that when she gave birth to her first child, my sister, Susan, the exquisite joy she felt bringing life into the world was trailed by a melancholy, the knowledge that her child would someday die. *Memento mori.*

In love we are vulnerable. We swoon, weak-kneed. We grow dizzy with yearning, ulceric with desire: *love-sick.* When I am in love I get an ache in my chest like I've been punched. But love's affliction is exquisite: attraction, flirtation, infatuation, passion. Love is the zenith: at the top, exaltation, vertigo. A fall. We *fall* in love. "There is hardly any activity, any enterprise, which is started with such tremendous hope and expectations," Erich Fromm wrote, "yet which fails so regularly as love." Falling in love has always come easily to me. It's the landing that is hard.

When I returned from backpacking in Europe, I bought a one-way ticket to Michigan. On the plane, I wore the same t-shirt I'd worn in nine countries, the one Steve had given me before I'd left, white italic letters on black cotton: *Someone misses me in Michigan.* I loved that Steve blazed his longing on this shirt, now on my body. But I was puzzled by the syntax. Shouldn't it have read, *Someone in Michigan misses me?* Steve's wording was an invitation, I concluded: he missed my presence *there*, in Michigan, where I never stepped foot until that July day in 1984.

My knees were wobbly as I disembarked in Detroit. I'd been apart from Steve as long as I'd known him—two months. Beardless and clean-shaven, wearing a striped jersey, Steve looked boyish, as if he'd grown younger in the months past. We hugged awkwardly, and I started toward the baggage claim. He stopped me. "Can I have a kiss?"

I smiled, and we fell into our blissful co-existence. We drove west toward the center of the state. From the cab of Steve's pickup truck, I could see everything, miles of dusty cornfields and laying-down buildings, squat architecture. In the New England landscape where I grew up, with twists and turns and hills and escarpments, you learned to be wary of what lurked around the bend. Southern Michigan's sheet-cake landscape didn't contain much of anything, which offered a sense of security. Then again, there was no place to hide. "It's so flat," I said.

Steve brought me to his four-bedroom house where he'd lived with his family. He'd moved them back to the first house he'd restored and had been renting, and put the larger house on the market. He couldn't afford the mortgage and a home for himself. The house was empty but for his bed in the walk-out basement, where it was cooler for sleeping. I walked through his kid's rooms but there was no evidence of them: no crayon marks on the walls, no tiny plastic doll shoe left behind, or bite marks on the window sills.

In the mornings Steve left for work, driving an hour to Ann Arbor to the union hall, then to various construction sites. I'd sleep late, then sprawl on the grass by the pond or on the couch in the damp basement, and read. Engrossed in *Lolita*, I passed hours in Nabokov's fictional world. My vice since childhood: the gluttony of reading, the delicious exile of books. When I'd finished reading the few books I'd packed (there were none in Steve's house—his favorite author, he said, was Dr. Seuss), I rode to Ann Arbor with him and dropped him off at the contractor's office. While he was at work, I'd buy a guest pass and swim a mile at the YMCA, and later peruse the musty used book stores. In the afternoon, I'd sit in the library and scan the employment section of the paper, which seemed pointless since I didn't know what I was qualified to do with my liberal arts degree, or even if I was staying in Michigan.

"What should I do?" I asked Steve nightly. Move to Michigan or return to Boston. Stay or go. Why was this so difficult? I must have sensed that the path I chose at this juncture would determine where I'd arrive in life. I must have intuited that choice is loss; by opting for one road, we forfeit the other. I was still young enough to want everything, to be both thrilled and terrified by the blank canvas of my life.

Indecision allows all possibilities to remain. Steve was no help, which was also no interference. It was my future, after all.

"You have to do what you want," he'd say.

"But do *you* want me to stay?"

"Only if *you* want to," he'd reply.

Trapped in a Mobius loop of ambivalence, I called my mother one night. "Just follow your heart," she said. Simple advice, cliché even, but she believed that the heart was a compass pointing true north. Everything seemed clear then: my heart was with Steve, and Steve was in Michigan.

Over Labor Day, Steve and I drove to Massachusetts to pack my possessions, which fit into the bed of his pickup truck. My father came over to the house I grew up in, and my mother and my four sisters and two brothers gathered to say goodbye.

"The Midwest is not that far," my father said. "You didn't cry when you said you might stay in Europe for a year." Everyone laughed.

"That was different," I said. The move to Michigan had an air of permanence about it, not a carefree backpacking trip, but the beginning of my adult life away from family and friends and everyone I knew.

"Michigan's not in the Midwest," Steve said. "It's in the same time zone as Massachusetts. It's practically on the east coast!"

I adored his hopeful revisionist geography, his rearranging of whole regions to accommodate me. Later, my father and Steve shook hands as they stood in the kitchen of my childhood home. "Take care of my daughter," my father said.

"I will," Steve promised.

"Hey," I said to them. "I can take care of myself."

When I heard my words declared aloud, I almost believed them.

Half-way across the country, at one o'clock in the morning, somewhere on a bumpy two-lane highway in western Pennsylvania, in the black of night, Steve and I argued, which surprised us both; we'd thought ourselves immune. I'm not sure how it started, but I remember the pith of it. "How do you think I felt when the first thing you asked your mother was if you got a letter from Bob? Or if Tim called?" Steve said. Bob was my pen-pal from college. We shared a love of books and writing. I'd had a crush on him, but he'd been an exchange student from the University of Oregon when we met and he'd returned there years before. Tim was a high school friend in whom I'd never had any romantic interest.

I was taken aback by Steve's jealousy, which he hadn't shown in New York nor in the letters he'd written to me while I was in Europe. Maybe I hadn't mentioned my friendships with Bob or Tim. They weren't my best friends, nor part of my daily life. Steve pulled the truck off the highway and parked in the shadowy lot of a closed gas station.

"Do you want to go back?" he asked.

"Of course not," I said. "Bob is just a friend. Would I leave my family behind and move halfway across the country if I didn't love you?" The more I insisted, the less convincing I sounded.

"You can still change your mind," he said. "I won't be mad, I just want you to be sure."

"I don't want to go back." I said. "Unless you don't want me here."

We were back in our circles, each of us perhaps hoping the other would halt our venture; each of us hoping that the other would be certain for both. We'd known each other only a matter of weeks. Our faith in love wavered for the moment, though neither of us wanted to admit that. We'd created in our minds a wonderful fantasy future, but maybe if we tried to transform the fantasy into reality, it would cease to be wonderful. We'd lose control of the perfect dream. Desire is forever *wanting*, not *having* (perhaps why so many marriages fail). But foregoing love for fear of its loss seemed cowardly. Love demands optimism. Or perhaps we'd come too far along the trajectory to stop ourselves. What force was necessary to turn a half-ton truck loaded with my life's possessions 180 degrees in the opposite direction? To backtrack the 600 miles we'd traveled after the dramatic, tearful departure in front of all my family?

On that still moonlit morning, half-way between my past and Steve's, on the verge of our future together, it must have seemed uncourageous to retreat. Instead, we disregarded our apprehensions, apologized, forgave each other. As if to reify our decision to remain united, we made love in the truck, the windows fogging from clouds we created with our warm quick breath, the stick shift jabbing into my leg, my head pressed against the dashboard, consummating our love in the truck's impossible space.

5. Love is Bountiful

On my backpacking trip across Europe, I'd visited my great aunts and uncles on my father's side, who lived in the unyielding rock-studded fields north of Galway, Ireland. Tough as sinew, they refused to succumb to poverty and harsh conditions, surviving to be eighty, ninety, a hundred years old. The palm reader I'd seen in London had predicted that I'd live to be eighty, like my great Uncle Sean with his glaucous eyes and ears like enormous rinds, tending three anemic cows. He lived in the thatched-roof stone hut he and my grandmother grew up in, still without electricity, heat, or plumbing in 1984. He spoke only Gaelic.

Places shape us. They forge our lexicon, how we dress, eat, think, the essence of our character, as if we are born from a mold cut from the stone of our birthplace, fed on the soil, contoured by the winds and the slant of light toward which we raise our faces. How is it that I felt more at home in Ireland where I'd only visited than I did in Michigan, a state in my own country? How did I lose myself knowing exactly where I was?

Saline, Michigan, twenty miles southwest of Ann Arbor. That's where Steve and I settled. Saline: I hated the name. Medicinal, like the saline solution injected into the uterus in second trimester abortions. Like the hometown I fled at eighteen, Saline was working class, with a huge Ford factory employing 4,000 people, a Ford dealership, a UAW union hall with a sign that read: *Parking for American Made Cars Only.*

In the town center were offices, a beauty parlor, sub shop, hardware store.

Steve and I rented the upstairs of a converted farmhouse a block from the town center. The apartment had blue shag carpeting in the bedroom, brown shag in the living room, dark paneled walls, and swirling lime-green linoleum in the kitchen. The only redeeming feature was a romantic alcove in the master bedroom, painted lavender and just large enough to fit Steve's queen-size bed. But the apartment was temporary; we intended to stay only long enough to save money for our dream home in the country.

Love is bountiful. If we chose to, we could allow the whole world into our hearts. Because I loved Steve, by extension I loved his children. Not long after I arrived in Michigan, Steve and I picked his kids up and drove them to Saline for the weekend. Nate and Lisa were quiet, but Sarah, the oldest, plunged into conversation. "I have Mrs. Connelly for third grade this year," she said. Of Steve's children, Sarah was most like him, bright and observant and forthright. Her coloring was exquisite: hair like flames, eyes gorgeously blue, fire and water. She had thick, blondish eyelashes and heavy lids like Steve's, which gave them both a sleepy look.

Lulled by the highway ride, Lisa fell asleep, her peach-colored dress bunching around the seat belt, exposing her doughy thighs. Her fluffy, caramel-colored hair was gathered into two awry pigtails, as if they'd been tacked on by blindfolded six-year-olds playing Pin-the-Tail-on-the-Donkey. With her hazel eyes, straight nose and long face, Lisa had inherited her mother's looks. Nate had white-blond, bone-straight flyaway hair, blue eyes sunk in a pudgy face, like a foam rubber boy, Pan's own son, with a pug nose. Nate was only four, but with his blunt, old-fashioned boy's haircut and worried expression, he seemed older. I craned my neck around and smiled at him in the back seat. He stared at me. "How come you have blue teeth?"

Steve glanced in the rear view mirror. "That's not nice, Nate," he said, and winked at me.

"That's okay," I said. "He's just being honest." That's what I love about kids; they keep you straight. You can hardly lie to yourself, let alone anyone else. I started to explain to Nate about my capped tooth, but he'd lost interest already, happily staring out the window at corn fields and combines and horses and cows. We pulled into the dirt parking lot of a VFW hall transformed into fair grounds. The kids rode the merry-go-round and a tiny Ferris wheel, ate snow-cones and hot dogs, rode a weary Shetland pony around a dinky circle of dirt. Nate held tightly to the reins, a bit frightened but determined. As he passed us, he'd lift one finger from his iron grip, a gesture at waving. Nate reminded me of myself at that age, a nervous, hand-wringing child.

Steve walked alongside the pony to support Lisa in the saddle, pulling his hanky from his back pocket like a magician's scarf to wipe her nose. Sarah rode the pony last, rolling her eyes as her horse trotted by; at eight, she was too mature to be amused. She and I were fast friends, especially after I let her wear my over-sized, burgundy-framed sunglasses. Sarah smiled for every snapshot like a movie star, with her pouty mouth and shiny orange hair, delicately eating pinches of pink cotton candy.

The pleasure of being with children is that you re-inhabit your own childhood. Resting on a bench between rides, I bounced Lisa on my lap in a game my father played with me. *Lisa went to Boston, Lisa went to Lynn. On the way to Boston, Lisa fell in.* I opened my knees and pretended to drop her through to the ground. She laughed and we played again. Later, we wandered between the rides and games and popcorn stands, Steve cradling Lisa in one arm, holding Nate's hand with his other. Sarah reached for my hand, which made me feel brave—her sticky palm clasped in mine—the way I'd felt when I was a teenager and I'd take my four-year-old brother Mikey down into the dark, scary basement to retrieve something from the freezer.

At a family gathering soon after, I met Steve's parents. Louise, his mother, was a petite blonde with pretty blue eyes behind cat-eye glasses. She had a precise manner, stepping lightly in her neatly ironed, coordinated blouse and shorts, a strained expression on her face. All day, she avoided me. Steve resembled his father, Bill, who was tall and lean, handsome still in his mid-fifties, though his hair was thinning across his tanned scalp. He seemed hapless in an endearing way, and kept busy grilling burgers, but he said hello and was friendly.

Steve's parents, conservative, church-going Lutherans, were wary of me, and frowned on Steve and I living together. After witnessing his troubled marriage, they didn't want him to make another calamitous choice. I didn't understand their cool reception. Couldn't they see that we were in love? Wasn't it obvious that I was Steve's true love, his first and only real love? Wouldn't any parents want that for their child above all else: love?

Steve introduced me to his sisters. Linda, who was two years younger, had curly blonde hair like Steve's and the family's crystalline blue eyes. She was pretty, with a ready, tinkling laugh; I admired her light spirit. She reminded me of my older sister, Sue, steady and grounded and kind-hearted. Linda's husband, Kevin, was friendly with country manners, and quick-witted. Kevin worked in a factory, a "shop rat," he called himself. Linda was a secretary. They'd been high school sweethearts. Karen, Steve's other sister, was a senior in high school, ten years younger than Steve. She was tall and lithe, with the family's enviable creamy skin, perfect white teeth, fair-haired, with prominent cheekbones that give her face an Asiatic cast.

I met cousins and aunts and uncles. The men stood in a circle telling off-color jokes, while the women prepared food or talked at picnic tables, keeping one eye on their children. This unnerved me, too, these traditional roles. Even the food made me feel like a stranger: opaque pink gelatin with shapes and objects floating in it; cold spaghetti saturated with salad dressing; package-mix blueberry muffins. Everything from recipes out of women's magazines, nothing like the food my mother cooked from scratch with real butter. Or the food I'd eaten in college, brown rice, tofu, alfalfa sprouts bloomed in a jar on my windowsill. Or the food that my sister Sally had recently introduced me to, dishes she prepared at her job as line chef at Chillingsworth on Cape Cod, where the Kennedys dined: grilled bluefish, lobster strudel, new potatoes glazed in aioli.

I'd always considered myself working class. My Italian grandmother was a maid, my Irish grandmother a cafeteria worker; one grandfather a groundskeeper, the other a forklift driver. My mother had a high school diploma, then went to vocational school for a nursing degree in her thirties after she and my father divorced. My father, with his master's degree, was the only son in his family to attend college. But Steve's family was a different sort of working class—less ambitious, it seemed to me then, contrary to my family's ethos. Or perhaps it was an east-coast snobbery that I was unaware I had, having never been to the Midwest until then. All day at Steve's parent's house I felt out of place, like a foreigner. All day I wished I hadn't worn the bright red, pointy-toed high-top sneakers I bought in Amsterdam, my thrift shop blouse, earrings I'd made of fishing lures. I barely ate, spoke to few of the adults, with whom, it appeared, I had little in common. Instead, I played with Sarah and Nate and Lisa, or hovered near Steve.

A kind of suffocating sadness washed over me whenever Steve and I drove to his hometown, as we did weekly to pick up his kids, and once a month on a Sunday to have dinner with his parents. In their economically-depressed manufacturing town, Steve's family struggled to make ends meet, suffering periodic lay-offs. Bill was a talented carpenter, his back slightly curved from the work, but he found employment only sporadically. They played euchre on weekends, fished in the summer, hunted in autumn. Nobody seemed to venture beyond Michigan too often.

They were happy, of course, I just couldn't see it. Their lives didn't fit the grand vision I had for myself. I understood, though, why Steve had escaped this town at eighteen, had vowed to never return. I understood why he fell in love with the mountains of Colorado, summits reaching beyond anything he'd ever seen, height instead of asphyxiating flatness: majesty over plainness. When Steve returned from Colorado to marry Deborah, he'd hired an artist to render in oils a photograph he'd shot in the Rockies: bluish-green spruce boughs in the foreground framing distant snow-capped peaks.

I wondered how Steve could bear to look at that painting, which hung in his parents' living room. It saddened me, knowing how things had turned out for him, the unhappy marriage, eight years of fighting, of working two jobs, taking classes at the local junior college to become an electrician, apprenticing for three years at minimum wage. Maybe for Steve the painting was not a symbol of what was forever lost, I thought, but what still could be.

One Sunday after dinner at Steve's parents' house, I met Joey, Steve's childhood friend. He'd noticed Steve's truck in the driveway and stopped to say hello. Joey and Steve shot pool in the basement. Joey wore dirty jeans, a beat-up leather jacket on his slight frame. He was balding, with a ring of brown hair brushing his shoulders. He reminded me of the townies I'd known, former high school athletes still hanging around the center, looking for parties, small-time drug dealers who never left, the high-school girls they enticed into their cars changing year after year. Joey worried me; perhaps I didn't really know Steve if he had friends like Joey.

Later that day, Steve, Joey and I perused their high school yearbook, Joey and I flanking Steve on the couch as we scanned rows of black and white portraits. They'd graduated in 1974 and so everyone's hair was mashed down. Steve looked handsome, even with plastered bangs rippling across his forehead and mutton-chop sideburns. Joey had a full head of hair, and the monochrome photography smoothed his acne-pitted skin. They looked so hopeful, those young strangers, the way the photographer positioned them looking up to the camera, guileless and naive, recording their dreams and aspirations. Steve touched the head shots of his classmates, pronouncing life sentences. Ten years had passed since they graduated, and people's fortunes could be told. "Divorced... divorced... in jail... dead."

We paused at the picture of the dead kid because it was strange that someone from high school had died already, only a decade later. I remember as a teenager having no sense of mortality, which was either not believing or sometimes not caring that I would die. In my twenties, I was less reckless with my life. But even confronted with evidence of the inevitable—the *fact* of death in black and white—I still felt, by virtue of youth, exempt.

6. A Tiny Dark Ship

a tiny dark ship is unmoored into the flow of the body's rivers...
Billy Collins, "Picnic, Lightning"

That fall, our first together, cells inside Steve's body multiplied rapidly, reproducing as quickly and efficiently as a factory assembly line. One by one the rogue cells embarked on journeys throughout Steve's body, traveling the network of veins in search of a place to light and continue their steadfast mission: replication, cells begat cells, fecundity and growth: life, though Steve's body was busy manufacturing death.

Inside my body, a similar process was taking place. Cells divided, multiplied. Halving begat doubling: mitosis, meiosis. In November of my first Michigan autumn, I began to vomit in the mornings. The flu, I thought, or possibly an anxious stomach. I developed an unusual craving for popsicles, something cold, something to bite. I bought huge boxes of assorted fruit-flavored popsicles, twenty-four to a box, and at night, wrapped in sweaters and blankets I'd eat three or four popsicles in a row, or five, or six.

When the morning nausea persisted, I made an appointment with a women's health center in Ypsilanti. The day my pregnancy was confirmed, I lied on our bed for hours, immobilized. Steve held me, but we didn't speak. Finally I said, "I have to schedule an abortion." I knew the circumstances were wrong; our relationship was fledgling; I hadn't found a job let alone a career; and Steve's divorce was not yet final. If

Steve had said, *I want us to have this baby*, perhaps I would have been persuaded to let a mistake alter the course of our lives. But he'd done that once already. "I'm sorry," he said. "My first marriage started this way and that turned out horribly. I want everything to be right for us." We'll have kids later, we agreed, after we were married.

On a Saturday, Steve drove me to the clinic for The Procedure, the euphemism the nurses used. He waited with me in the lounge while I grew woozy from a painkiller. And then I was on a gurney flat on my back with my knees bent and thighs spread, my head floaty from drugs, a nurse holding my hand while a doctor dilated my cervix with progressively larger wands, then tidily vacuumed my uterus of blood and tissue and the tiny zygote that Steve and I had accidentally ignited.

Afterward, outside in the parking lot of the clinic, Steve gave me a present: a stereo system for our car. I knew he meant well, bless his heart, meant to give me something I'd wanted, something expensive, but I was too sad to appreciate his gesture. I slept the rest of the day, and sulked for a week. I opened the freezer but had no trace of desire for the popsicles, which I threw in the garbage. I realized that I had to *do something*, make something happen, make my life. Nobody was going to do that for me. I signed up with four temporary employment agencies, and renewed my efforts to find a job, any job.

Quickly my life in Michigan failed to live up to my expectations, though I wasn't even sure what my expectations were. I hadn't envisioned this life I'd chosen, hadn't put any rational thought into my decision to move here and live with Steve. Each morning I fixed Steve's lunch, kissed him goodbye, which felt so conventional. I napped until 9:00 a.m. or so, then circled jobs in the classifieds. I thought my bachelor's degree was something special and would land me a job like those I sent resumes for: marketing manager, staff writer, public relations officer. I'd clean the apartment, then had long empty hours until Steve returned. I wrote "to do" lists in my journal, recorded dreams, ideas for free-lance articles: *article on creative fighting—use techniques of mediation.* This idea was not conceived for Steve and me, but for he and Deborah whose divorce was contentious. After one altercation in Deborah's driveway with Steve yelling and Deborah kicking Steve's car, the neighbors called the cops. From then on, the court ordered Deborah to remain in her house and Steve to stay his car when he picked up the kids on weekends. It was heartbreaking to see little Lisa dragging her tiny heavy suitcase down the steps and across the driveway.

In my journal I captured stray thoughts and sentences, which seem nonsensical now: *Steps come from the felt edge. To dance is to hold a meteor shower starring the toe.* I conversed with myself: *What is freedom? What is aloneness? What is loneliness?* I tried to write short stories but felt enervated, so instead I watched soap operas. The soaps were a fix; they kept me pinned to the couch for three hours straight, hypnotized by characters and their faulty lives filled with bad decisions and rash actions that lead only to trouble. In soap operas, time passed slowly, the same problems cropping up day after day with only incremental changes, characters who never aged.

But soap opera time felt fleeting to me, turning day into night economically, Steve pulling into the driveway just as the last show ended and it was time to cook supper. Saline, Michigan might as well have been Port Charles from *General Hospital* or Pine Valley from *All My Children*, I felt that removed from my life. Michigan felt foreign to me, like the countries I visited in Europe, but familiar enough that I didn't understand why I felt alienated. In Saline, that conservative Midwestern hamlet, I began to lose a grip of who I was.

In wintertime, frogs estivate; they sink to the bottom of the pond, nestle into mud and slow their breathing to survive on minimal oxygen. Barely alive, they wait out the cold. That's how I felt after the crisp October days turned cold and gray in November, then December. The grayness of Michigan's skies, caused by the "lake effect," lingered for weeks, a uniform canvas: no texture, no relief. I cried every night. Steve tried desperately to cheer me up. Each night he brought home a little gift: a chocolate bar, a silly card, odd items like emery boards or a pair of tweezers (I must have mentioned needing them). One day he presented me with a branch of pussy willow glazed with ice that he'd found on his work site and saved in the back of his truck all day. The little fuzzy cat's-paw buds shimmered brilliantly before melting.

But as the weeks passed, Steve lost faith in his ability to please me, which only sharpened my despair, Steve working so hard to cheer me up, knowing in my heart his efforts were futile, that my sadness had little to do with him. I couldn't name these bouts of melancholy yet; I wouldn't know for years that my grandmother, my father, and my sister suffered depression, too. I assured Steve that I would be fine, everything would be fine, I just needed to get a job, to adjust. "I know you miss your family," he said, offering to pay for a flight to Boston. But they were the *last* people I wanted to see, those who cared too much for my happiness, who were waiting, holding their breath, to see if everything would work out for me in Michigan, my first real venture into my own life.

One day, Sho-Pro Windows called. I'd left an application in their office weeks earlier. I interviewed, took an hour-long personality test ("Would you rather be a forest ranger or an airplane pilot," etc.), and was hired, my only job offer. In three weeks of sales training, I learned the seven-step method to sell the deluxe, vinyl-clad, triple-paned, steel-reinforced replacement windows. At night, I practiced my demonstration for Steve, who sat on the couch and posed difficult questions, or acted impossibly ignorant and silly. I sprayed Freon on the outside of the sample window until a thermometer registered zero and like a magician, pointed to a second thermometer on the inside pane, which read a comfortable room temperature. Steve applauded.

I drove to sales calls on evenings and weekends, spending hours with potential customers, who were typically working-class couples in generic ranch houses in the grid of Detroit's suburbs: Warren, Romulus, Sterling Heights, which was completely flat—"height" a term for the economic aspirations of its residents. I inspected the couple's windows, pointing out damaging condensation, rotted sills, and—worst of all—windows painted shut. We'd been instructed to spin a story about a possible fire, the inability to escape because of stuck windows, broken glass, blood, smoke, suggestions of calamity and loss.

But I couldn't or wouldn't push expensive windows using this scary tale; perhaps that was why for a month I didn't sell a single window. Meanwhile, my coworkers were earning commissions. Their histograms—charts in which bars reach higher and higher like skyscrapers—were rising. My bar resembled the squat ranch houses of my would-be clients. Meanwhile, Steve was miserable. He grumbled when I left the house on Saturday mornings in my cheap polyester suit, carrying a fake-leather briefcase that I bought at K-Mart for twelve dollars. "I miss you," he'd say.

Finally, one night I sold one window to a couple whose budget after bills contained the exact payment for a single, super-deluxe "Cadillac of windows." The husband earned ten dollars an hour in a supermarket. The wife was a stay-at-home mother to their three children. At midnight, just after I closed the deal, the husband said to his weary wife, "We'll put it in the baby's room." He turned to me, "There's a terrible draft in there."

I felt awful taking this couple's last spare income, yet I'd followed the seven steps and the process had worked. At home, I told Steve the news.

"You have to quit that job or we're through," he said. He must have feared that my taste of success would lure me further away from him, but that was not the kind of reception I'd expected upon my first sale.

"You can't just issue an ultimatum," I said.

"That crummy job is more important than us? We never see each other. How is that a relationship?" It *was* a crummy job, but it was *my* crummy job, my first white-collar job after college, not dead-end bartending. "You hate that job anyway," Steve said. "And you don't make any money." This was true, but his comment only emphasized my failure.

It was two a.m. when the argument ended, mostly out of exhaustion. The next morning I sat in my boss's office and, slobbery with tears, resigned. I couldn't lift the sample window out of my trunk (on sales calls, I'd ask the husbands for help), so instead of slinking away after quitting, I was forced to shuffle back into my boss's office and ask him to retrieve the window. Driving home, I felt weightless and giddy, glad that Steve had provided me with an excuse to quit that loathsome job. But underneath my freedom, something nagged.

I worked temporary jobs for a month—switchboard operator for General Motors, bank receptionist, secretary—before I was hired as an administrative assistant in a small cottage business owned by Phyllis Nash, who ran a gift import business. In late January 1985, a fresh new year, I started working in Phyllis's basement office. My pay was $5.50 an hour with no benefits, half what I'd earned bartending at the Hitching Post. Besides myself and Phyllis, Maggie, a college student, worked part-time as a shipping clerk. Phyllis's maid, Peg, worked upstairs, polishing silver, cleaning stained glass windows, preparing gourmet meals from recipes Phyllis selected, *boudin* one day, which smelled savory and delicious, onions sautéed in butter and fresh thyme.

Most of my days were spent alone in Phyllis's dank basement, answering the telephone, processing orders. There was a fireplace in the room (and sometimes a fire). My spirits began to lift. I signed up for an evening drawing class and researched graduate programs, and finally winter released its grip on Michigan, which was not the Arctic Circle after all, and daylight yawned into the night, and down coats were stored, and shades of green unfurled all around, huge flags of lawns and leaves like confetti. I felt buoyed. My life had begun finally, at twenty-four. I felt like I was marching in a parade, spinning my baton down Main Street as I had in third grade, me going places, twirling. Steve and I were happy again, as if our love were weather dependent. We spent weekends exploring the countryside searching for an old farmhouse to buy. This was my first full summer in Michigan and the landscape was plush and verdant, ripe with offerings. We picked a half-bushel of strawberries at a U-Pick farm and ate them until we were sick with sweetness. We aged two gallons of strawberry wine in our bedroom closet, having no access to a cool cellar. In July, we plucked a bushel of tomatoes at a farm in Ypsilanti and canned dozens of quarts, all day in our kitchen dunking tomatoes in boiling water, then plunging them in an ice bath, peeling skins, quartering and salting—our fingers raw from the extremes of temperature—then stuffing mason jars, loading them in the pressure-cooker for forty-five minutes, removing the hot bottles with tongs and stocking our pantry, preserving against the possibility of scarcity.

One Saturday Steve and I purchased a used ice-cream maker at a yard sale. The kids were excited as we filled the canister with warmed cream and sugar and vanilla bean, set the bucket in our bathtub packed with rock salt. We took turns cranking the antiquated machine for an arm-deadening hour. While we waited for the ice cream to freeze, Sarah and I strung bead necklaces. She played dress-up with my clothes, the outlandish garb I rarely wore anymore in Saline, clomping around the house in my fuchsia suede Peter Pan-style boots.

I taught her to type on my second-hand word processor. She named her file, "Blue Moon," the title of a sad ballad, her life at age nine. (Five years older than her next sibling, Sarah had witnessed more of the turmoil of her parents' marriage.) Lisa watched cartoons. Nate asked for help drawing an airplane. I loved Nate's little form, his miniature Buddha belly and puffy, saxophonists'-inflated cheeks. Nate was stocky, not slender and long like Steve, but like a Labrador puppy with too-big hands and feet. He reminded me of a gingerbread boy. Risen, lopsided, sweet.

I drew an airplane and he tried to copy my figure, but couldn't keep his lines straight. Frustrated, he began to cry. I showed him again, but he failed each time. "It takes practice, Nate," I said, feeling as if I'd done something wrong, violated some parenting rule about drawing better than the child. Steve had been a parent at nineteen, so he had nine years of practice already. He picked up Nate and wiped his eyes, asked him if he wanted to try the home-made ice cream. Steve ladled three bowls of soupy vanilla.

"How is it Nate?" I asked.

"It's cold and good," he said, like a line of haiku. I felt that there was poetry in our lives, and beauty. At dusk one weekend night, we took the kids to the park in Saline for a hot air balloon festival. The evening was too windy for the balloons to launch, but we were thrilled watching the enormous colorful pouches three stories high inflate and undulate in the breeze like huge tropical jellyfish, straining to break free of their tethers, the roar of the gas flame lending them voice and anima.

At night, Steve bathed Lisa and Nate, carefully lathering their scalps, mindful not to drip soap in their eyes. He gently combed out the tangles in Lisa's waist-length hair, fastened plastic poodle barrettes to fetter the wispy strands. He snapped them into their one-piece, footed pajamas like little astronauts ready for take-off. Pajama time was crazy time. The kids spent the last of their energy like the grand finale of a fireworks display. We danced around the living room to Steve's Bob Seger tapes, while Steve entertained us with his silly walk: a kind of dip and bounce, pretending to be a rock star, exaggeratedly mouthing lyrics to his favorite song, Seger's "Turn the Page." We feasted on Steve's home-made cheese popcorn, watched a rented movie, and one by one the kids fell asleep in their sleeping bags on the living room floor, those puffy perfect faces and tiny warm bodies that migrated toward each other in sleep, seeking warmth and comfort, like a huddle of gerbils.

In the morning, we heard the kids stirring, breathing at our doorknob, willing the door open with their raspy breath like the wolf in the "Three Little Pigs." Sleepy-eyed and gnarly-haired, Lisa burst through the door, sent as an envoy by Sarah and Nate who knew better than to enter without knocking. Once the door was open, Nate and Sarah followed. "Can we watch cartoons?" Steve rose and asked the kids what they wanted for breakfast. Nate wanted scrambled eggs. Sarah, with her sweet tooth, favored pancakes. Steve cooked, while I lounged in bed.

On those weekends we were a little family, and I was happy. I enjoyed the regression of playing with the kids, their bodied presentness, their unfiltered needs, feelings explicitly expressed. Hunger, fatigue, frustration, delight. For a long time, I'd thought that Shakespeare had written, "To thy *known* self be true" — instead of "To thine *own* self be true." But the former seemed more fitting to me. Being with the kids restored me to my *known* self, not someone I was trying to be, or thinking I should become, some mature, adult person who was not silly, not moody, not selfish or insecure.

On Sunday afternoons, after we dropped the kids back home, I'd sit in front of a full-length mirror and draw myself, the weekly assignment for my class. At first, my drawings were loose and wild, one eye larger than the other, with a long, thin neck that was not mine. A common mistake in beginning portraiture is to draw your eyes too large, as if observing yourself for hours has a magnifying affect. Studying my own external image—learning about perspective and shape and shadow—forced me to examine my interior self, as if the mirror revealed layers of identity, not just the surface.

Week after week, as my portraits began to resemble me more closely, I noticed a correlation between my push outward in the world and increased tension with Steve. He began to draw an invisible circle around me, first requesting that I stop writing to my college friend Bob. I needed Bob to discuss books and films and art, subjects about which Steve wasn't conversant. "Bob's three thousand miles away," I said. "Can't you believe that I have no desire for anyone else?"

Steve didn't believe that men and women could have Platonic friendships. I acquiesced; I stopped writing to Bob. He and I exchanged only a few letters a year, so waning to none seemed more like a hiatus, I rationalized, not an end. But Steve was still insecure. Afraid of losing me, he reigned me in. "Don't ever leave me, Mo," he said one day. "I won't," I said, which was only partially dishonest. I had no plans to leave Steve; I hoped to marry him. But I secretly reserved that choice in case I fell out of love. That was how I viewed love then, as a fatalistic force over which I had no control, like falling from a bunk bed, which I'd done as a child.

Within everything exists the kernel of its own destruction. As months passed, the affection and adoration Steve gave me, the love and attention I'd thrived on began to smother me. He grew increasingly jealous, one day accusing me of flirting with the bag boy at the supermarket, another time with a man at the lake where we'd picnicked. Our fight about that accusation spilled over into the evening, half-teasing, half-arguing, neither of us willing to capitulate. Steve thought I was a flirt; I thought he was delusional. Steve did not see himself as insecure, stubborn, and controlling. I did not see myself as uncompromising, stubborn, and controlling. We saw fault only in the other.

I didn't understand that my romantic history worried Steve (compared to his lack of same), that he thought I'd just leave him when someone else came along; he worried someone else *would* come along. "I don't know why you're with me," he said sometimes. I thought Steve should just trust me *a priori*, that I shouldn't have to earn his trust. I didn't understand the basis of his fears, or how to reassure him of my fidelity, my commitment. Maybe he didn't trust me because he sensed that I was withholding something, which I was: that if I no longer loved him, I *would* leave him. But this was a self-fulfilling prophecy: the more he didn't trust me, the more he saw my actions as suspect, the more I wanted to break away from him. Our recurring argument was eroding our foundation of happiness. I began to see that he and I were becoming just that—*he* and *I*, no longer *us*.

7. Paddle

If there is one thing one can always yearn for, and sometimes attain, it is human love.
— Albert Camus, *The Plague*

S teve and I had attained love; we just couldn't hold fast to it. After that fight, I asked Steve to see a couple's counselor, but he refused. Instead we took a vacation, which I thought would be a panacea, time alone to patch up our relationship: a geographic tonic. Steve was tired, and his back ached, which we attributed to his physically demanding job. He'd been working ten hour shifts, often six days a week for nearly a year, saving money to buy a house so that the kids could live with us in summers. He'd finally won joint custody in his divorce settlement.

Steve bought a second-hand camper for $600, a 1968 pistachio-green pop-up with no refrigerator or bathroom, not much more than glorified tent. We spent a weekend scrubbing it inside and out, then headed north. Hours later, on a spit of land under the Mackinac Bridge, a five-mile suspension bridge at the Straits of Mackinac where Lakes Michigan and Huron couple, huddled in sweatshirts against the autumn chill, Steve and I sat in our chaise longues and stared at the span, which looked suspended on faith alone, a feat of engineering we marveled at until sundown, drinking our strawberry wine, a pulpy brownish liquid heavily dosed with Mountain Dew, which only incrementally improved the acrid swill. But it was *our* swill, mashed and sieved and strained and filtered, then aged for months, so we drank it and liked it. Steve seemed relaxed and happy.

The next day we ventured to Michigan's northernmost reaches toward the shores of Lake Superior. The single lane highway was like a tunnel through conifer forest with few stores or houses or traffic lights. The landscape was crowded with miles of balsam fir, sweeping white pines, and tamaracks, but unpeopled; it felt stark and lonely. We stopped at Tahquamenon Falls, the second most voluminous falls in the country, and walked along the fenced trail a hundred feet above the roiling Tahquamenon River, eye-level with the edge where torrents of tannin-yellowed water rush over a cliff.

The park had few visitors in autumn, so nobody saw Steve climb over the split rail fence, past the warning signs where he could no longer hear me say, "Come back. Be careful. You're not supposed to be there." He climbed down the steep embankment to a ledge and watched the force of water tumbling. I snapped a photo of him, a long shot because I dared go no closer. His hair was unruly and long, neglected because of the time spent working. He held a cigarette between two fingers as he squatted on the precipice, courting danger. One slip of his foot and he'd be flotsam. I have another photo of Steve walking atop a four-inch wide railing, a thirty foot drop on one side. I admired his body-confidence, his proprioceptivity, his sure-footed feline grace, but these dare-devil feats worried me.

We made camp in a sunny spot on a tributary of the Tahquamenon, and then began blowing up the two-person rubber raft I'd ordered from a catalog. The tributary was knee high in places, but elsewhere was dark and deep and cold. Steve and I paddled under the creamy October sun, moving peacefully with the current until at some moment we realized that our vessel was losing air. The rubber raft was perfect for floating lazily, but a single muscular dip of my plastic oar didn't advance the boat, especially against the force of the current, which was away from our camp site.

"Paddle! Paddle!" Steve joked, and there was a sense of adventure and hilarity, until I calculated that even with the combined force of

Steve's strength and mine, the rate of the air hissing out of the raft was faster than the distance we gained. If we didn't take some other course of action, we'd swamp. I plunged my oar into the chilly water, but it didn't touch bottom. The tributary had carried us into the middle of a lake. I'd taken a junior lifesaving class when I was fourteen, so I knew how easy it was to drown. I envisioned the boat capsizing. I envisioned us being carried away in frigid water. I envisioned hypothermia and drowning and death.

Steve laughed. "It's not funny," I urged. "We're in danger. Paddle!"

Steve didn't worry much; I fretted enough for both of us. Somehow we made it to shore.

I picked up my book. Steve visited our neighbors across the way, a retired couple, Ken and Edna Davis from Three Rivers, Michigan— so announced on a wood-burned plank mounted on their Winnebago. Steve learned of a fishing spot from Ken Davis, so the next morning we drove to a road off Lake Superior's shore and hiked through woods along a shallow creek. Steve waded into the creek in rubber boots. I was content to watch as he cast his line into the sun-dappled water. The last time I fished—with my father when I was eight—I caught a catfish, but I couldn't bear to watch the creature gasping for breath, its jaw scissoring desperately, gills expanding, heaving and suffering. I'd started to cry, so my father quickly unhooked the fish and threw it back in the water.

The stream was replete with chubby foot-and-a-half long grayish coho salmon wending against the current with the last of their energy, intent, driven, pausing in eddies to lay eggs. I watched females hover in the shallow pools close to the banks, scoop dimples in the sand with their pelvic fins. And then at some moment when the female knew the cradle of sand was perfect, when some instinctual trigger clicked, she ejaculated orange beads the size of small pearls. The male coho, who'd been lurking nearby, swam over the eggs and released milky sperm, which clouded the water momentarily before the milt washed away in the current. The male's job seemed a haphazard affair, like tossing confetti on a windy day and hoping it landed in the exact right place: a foolhardy, scattershot approach, a last gesture toward life before it ended.

And then the fish ceased swimming, simply let themselves drift downstream with the flow, a gentle ride through the woods, under the overpass and into the greatest of lakes, Superior, a vast blue-gray basin. Fish heaven. Life and death within seconds of each other, conception cycling around mortality, pure biology.

Steve fished. Or it looked that way. He didn't tempt the fish with a juicy worm or delicate, surface-skimming fly. He simply cast a large, thumb-sized treble hook *at* the fish, hoping a barb would catch on the creature's mouth or tail or fin. Snagging fish seemed as primitive and potentially fruitless an approach as the male salmon's spawning effort. But the stream was swarming with fish and so this random, hit or miss method was eventually—arithmetically—successful. Steve hauled in six salmon, the smallest a foot long. He strung them on a rope, and I clicked a dozen photos: Steve with his catch hung on a line like laundry; Steve cleaning the fish; Steve and the biggest salmon. He had a cigarette in one hand, wore a magenta and blue striped jersey underneath his white cardigan, the one he'd worn the night we met at the Hitching Post, though now the sweater was misshapen and holey. He had two days of reddish stubble on his cheeks and wild uncombed hair. He smiled broadly, eyes squinted, dimples showing.

Steve delivered two big fish to Ken and Edna. Back at our camp he squeezed the roe from the females by pressing on the underbelly, then filleted the fish, smoking a cigarette, relaxed and businesslike. I shook the fillets in a brown paper sack with flour and salt and pepper and sautéed them in butter. The fish cooked up tender and white, every bite sweet and succulent. We drank our strawberry wine and lounged in our chaise longues looking at tiny, faraway stars, fiery bodies alive to us but who knows, perhaps extinguished already.

On our last night, Steve and I ate dinner with Ken and Edna Davis from Three Rivers, Michigan, sat with them awhile at their fire, then inside their luxurious camper with its microwave oven and television. Steve and Ken and Edna posed for a picture, Steve with his arm around Edna's shoulders, she hugging his waist, as if they were the best of friends, or even relatives. She could be his mother or at least his aunt. Edna's other arm linked through her husband's and they all three smiled, Steve, and Ken and Edna. We made a pact to meet on that very same date in October two years hence, when the salmon would spawn again. "We'll be here," Steve promised, and we all shook hands.

Back then, Steve and I worried that Ken and Edna wouldn't make the trip, older and nearer to the end of their lives as they were. Now when I see this picture, I envision Ken and Edna Davis in Tahquamenon Falls State Park, sitting in folding chairs outside their camper, wondering if we are coming, watching for us, waiting.

8. Thy Known Self

The next month, November, 1985, a year and a half after I moved to Saline, my sister, Sally, called to say she was relocating to Michigan. She'd been living in a tent for months, staked out in a campground on Cape Cod. Sally's move to Michigan was not as arbitrary as it seemed. She is an artist, and for years we vowed to live near each other, to collaborate on projects. In college, I starred in Sally's sixteen-millimeter film. She shot one scene on a frigid February morning, the air in the Berkshires dry and cold, white sun reflecting harshly off the ice of a forest pond. The woods were quiet but for great wracking groans from the ice contracting as it melted, the sound rising and vibrating in the still air. It was hauntingly beautiful, the ice breaking out of itself, moving like a living thing, toward liquid, toward air, another incarnation altogether.

For the scene, I was naked. My hot breath had turned to vapor, my words almost visible. "How fast should I run?" I asked Sally. I was to dart through the thick bramble, pushing branches out of my way, ignoring the scratches on my legs and arms that were more than verisimilitude. When I reached the edge of the pond, I knelt down on my hands and knees and looked around warily, like a hunted animal. I never asked Sally what she had in mind with this scene. I understood she had a vision, she was making art. I shivered. I ran.

When I told Steve that Sally was moving to Michigan, he said, "Good. She can live here because I'm moving out." In spite of our problems, which the vacation had not resolved, I was shocked by Steve's words.

"Please don't leave," I said. "I think we can work things out." Deep down I knew that our relationship was faltering, but I wanted to hang on because I loved Steve.

Over the next two weeks, Steve came home late from work, telling me that he'd been looking at apartments. Nightly I pleaded with him to reconsider. I hadn't resigned myself to his leaving, but Sally's arrival triggered a shift in me. When I saw my sister for the first time in nearly a year, I recognized in her vibrant spirit reflections of myself, essential elements that I'd let fall along the road to Michigan, like the mufflers and tailpipes and tires in the breakdown lane on the highway. In the year or so that I lived with Steve, I hadn't swam at the Y, I hadn't seen a foreign film or visited an art gallery. I hadn't written any stories. I'd traded my night time reading for snuggling with Steve on the couch, watching television. For comfort and safety, for love, I'd opted for passivity, for a circumscribed world. I was living Steve's idea of a life, not mine.

To thy *known* self be true. I chose to leave.

Steve did not ask me to stay, but after his surprise at my announcement, his silence and withdrawal signaled anger. Meanwhile, Sally and I found a tiny but charming apartment in Whitmore Lake, a bedroom community north of Ann Arbor. The apartment was the second story of a farmhouse at the end of a dirt road. We had two bedrooms, with a wood stove in the living room and a deck overlooking a small pond. I liked the sound of my new address—11505 Dunleavy Lane—alliterative and lyrical, with hints of noir, as in *Murder on Dunleavy Lane*, like the mystery stories Sally and I loved to read and write in childhood.

But I didn't spend many nights at Dunleavy Lane. Steve called me after two days. "I miss you," he said. I missed him, too, and so I visited him in Saline. He was having acute back pain then, which seemed to double in intensity each day. Often near tears, he begged me to give him back rubs so he could sleep at night. I began to spend most of my nights with Steve, stopping by Dunleavy Lane for clean clothes. From the empty beer bottles next to the refrigerator and the stack of videos waiting to be returned, I could see that Sally arrived home from her job, assistant chef at The Moveable Feast, drank beer, and watched movies.

That winter Michigan had a spell of cloudy days. Nearly a month passed without sun. (A sunny day, finally, was cause for a front-page headline in *The Detroit News*.) Sally had sunk into a pall of loneliness, immersed in vintage black and white films, which mimicked the colorlessness of Michigan's sky. I felt guilty for neglecting my sister, guilty for leaving Steve (after promising I *never* would). In my worst moments, I wished Sally would snap out of her funk, and at times I thought that Steve was malingering to keep me by his side. It seemed impossible that his back could ache so badly when he'd been seeing a chiropractor. But the pain persisted.

Finally, after a night when Steve was in excruciating agony, I grew alarmed. "You'd better go see a specialist. An internist or someone. Please."

January 28, 1986 was bitterly cold. I sat in a swivel chair that morning in Phyllis's basement office, warming my feet with a space heater. I was alone. Peg, Phyllis's housekeeper, hadn't arrived yet, so there were no quick sneaker-steps above me, no savory smells from the kitchen wafting down the stairs. It was quiet, except for the click click of the keyboard as I prepared invoices, and the radio in the background tuned to classical music. Then the regular programming on the radio station was cancelled to broadcast the launch of the space shuttle Challenger. As I listened to the countdown—nine, eight, seven—I had a thought so sudden and clear it seemed like a transmission: *they are going to die.*

I stopped typing. Two. One. They're off, the announcer exclaimed, this historic crew—seven astronauts and one schoolteacher, Krista

McAuliffe from New Hampshire. But wait, something happened. The Challenger exploded in mid-air, two vertiginous plumes of smoke. I couldn't see this; I could only hear the announcer's astonished voice as he described the tragedy. The hair on my arms prickled, and I felt guilty for my prescient thought, as if I'd somehow willed the explosion. And then I was crying, sitting alone in Phyllis's clammy basement, unsure of why I was sobbing, sensing perhaps that the loss of those lives was somehow my loss, too.

Three days later, I sat at the same desk distractedly sorting through the morning's mail, preoccupied still with the Challenger disaster, unnerved by the tragedy. How awful. How strange. Krista McAuliffe, one day a mother, a beloved teacher, ordinary. Suddenly an astronaut, a hero. The next day, vanished.

The phone rang. It was Steve. He'd gone to an orthopedist that morning for his back pain, a specialist who treated the University of Michigan's elite athletes.

"The doc wants me to check into the hospital," he said. He sounded calm, but this news made me anxious.

"When?" I asked.

"Right now," he said.

The doctor didn't allow Steve to drive home for a change of clothes or toiletries, so I promised to bring these after work. I said goodbye, trying to sound unworried. But after I hung up, my chest felt numb. My body filled with a diffuse sense of dread that seemed to have bled into my life from the Challenger disaster.

In my memory, these sensations are fused: the image of the Challenger exploding, the shrill jangle of the phone ringing, and my heart beating faster and faster.

PART II

9. Flintstones Chewables

What can happen in six hours? At work I'd earn $33, enough for dinner out. If I drove from Ann Arbor, I could reach another state, another nation entirely if I aimed northeast. Six hours can yield very little: one meal, or an entirely new country, Canada. In the six hours since Steve's phone call, he traveled only a short distance—two floors in St. Joseph's Hospital—but landed in new terrain altogether. That morning, Steve had suffered the nuisance of back pain. By dinner, he'd been moved to the oncology floor with its grim practitioners, Dr. Demmons, a tall, fortyish, imperious man with glasses and thick black hair, and Dr. Lin, a tiny, laconic Korean in her mid-fifties.

For days, the doctors ran tests: nuclear scans of Steve's skeleton, Magnetic Resonance Imaging, which outlined organs and nerves and muscles; upper and lower gastrointestinal x-rays to expose his digestive tract. I called my mother each night from Steve's room, where I slept on a cot next to his bed. A licensed practical nurse, she worked at a hospital in our hometown that specialized in cancer, the first in the country to do so. She speculated that Steve had Hodgkin's disease, a cancer of the lymphatic system that strikes young men more than women, usually in their late twenties and early thirties. Hodgkin's had an 80% survival rate. We prayed that Steve had Hodgkin's.

Four days after Steve was admitted to St. Joseph's, I had an interview for the position of Public Relations Manager of the Washtenaw Country Red Cross, which I'd scheduled weeks earlier. I wanted to cancel the interview, but Steve convinced me to follow through. "It's a good opportunity," he said, "a big step up in responsibility and salary."

I stayed at Sally's the night before the interview, ironing my suit, inspecting my nylons for runs, tossing and turning on a narrow squishy air mattress. The next morning, Sally's junker car stalled in the slushy mud-snow as she backed out of the driveway. I tugged on my boots to help her dislodge her monstrous, boxy Chrysler, then sped to my interview. I noticed the director of the Washtenaw County Red Cross staring at my feet as I sat in his office with my legs daintily crossed, realizing then that I'd forgotten my pumps back at the apartment. I fussed with the hem of my navy pin-stripe skirt, as if that would somehow hide the clunky, mud-caked boots. I noticed then the general disorder of my appearance, stray threads on the cuffs, a loose button, my faux-leather briefcase, which could not have fooled anyone; it was what it was, fake and cheap, like my coordinated sky-blue rayon blouse.

I considered making a joke about the boots, telling the story of my sister's car, but I was too unstable to natter on amusingly. Emotionally, I was zippered up for the interview. If I opened the portal for one emotion—laughter, even polite fake laughter—other emotions would surge out. I envisioned myself weeping sloppily while the perplexed director looked on aghast. I forced a smile, but the tinny flat voice that gamely answered the director's questions was not mine. It belonged to a persona, one as synthetic as my skirt and blazer, one shamelessly trying to advance her career while her boyfriend was in the hospital with cancer.

On Sunday, Bill and Louise brought the kids for a visit to St. Joe's. Lisa and Nate operated the remote control to raise and lower Steve's bed as if it were a carnival ride. They wandered up and down the halls, drank soda through straws, marveled at the tiny toy cars in the parking lot six stories below. I snapped a photo of Nate and Lisa on Steve's hospital bed, Lisa in braids fastened with yellow barrettes, wearing a flowered dress with puffy sleeves. Nate wore a short-sleeved, button-down white shirt and creased khaki pants, like a miniature man, all dressed up and smiling, enjoying the visit to the hospital as if it were an outing to the museum.

Sarah was uncharacteristically quiet. She was shy about sitting on Steve's bed or coming close to him. Maybe she noticed his pale complexion, the grayish smudges under his eyes already, like the priest's thumbprint on Ash Wednesday. Perhaps she intuited the seriousness of the situation; she was a perceptive child. Or maybe she was wondering about how—with her father in the hospital—we would celebrate her birthday in two weeks, when she'd turn ten.

After six days, Steve was still undiagnosed. Dr. Demmons and Dr. Lin were avoiding us; it wasn't my imagination. One night around midnight, a day or so after the doctors biopsied Steve's liver (inserting a cartoonish jumbo needle to draw out liver cells), I cornered an intern in the hallway and demanded to know the results of the tests. "I really can't say." The intern, a skinny young woman around Steve's age, looked frightened. Probably she detected an air of desperation about me.

"We've been here a week," I said. "Steve's had a half-dozen tests. You *must* know something. I mean, we know he has cancer. Where did it originate? Has it metastasized? What stage is it?" I had taken a course called Microbiology of Cancer in college to fill a science requirement, though I never imagined that this was how I'd put my college education to use. I wanted this intern and the other doctors to know that I was educated, unlike Steve and his parents, whom the doctors spoke to in simplistic terms, patronizing. Dr. Demmons demonstrated peristalsis to Steve's parents using a paper bag, as if he were speaking to an audience of fourth graders.

"You *have* to tell us," I pressed the intern. She understood that I was not going to let her walk away, that I would block her path, grab her white lab coat, follow her into the ladies room, the doctor's lounge.

"His cancer is widespread," she said. "That's all that I can say. It's not my job." She stepped around me and strode quickly down the hall.

The intern must have written a note on Steve's chart because the next day Dr. Lin came into Steve's room, leaned against the heater unit underneath the window, hands shoved deep into the pockets of her knee-length lab coat. "Steven," she said. "Your cancer is terminal. Unfortunately, there is no treatment. I'm very sorry. There's nothing we can do." She stood, patted Steve's hand, and walked out of the room.

We were shocked, not so much by her words, which we couldn't fully absorb (his *cancer* was terminal, she'd said, as if it were the disease that would end), but by the quickness and casualness with which she'd delivered the news, and her rapid exit. Steve cried a little, an impoverished, dry weeping. We hugged, but since we didn't really believe the prognosis, we did not forfeit ourselves to great sobbing. By the time Dr. Demmons visited later, we were prepared with questions. Steve had adenocarcinoma, Dr. Demmons told us. "It's a very aggressive type of cancer, in stage IV already. It probably started in the liver and has spread to the bones."

Steve was in bed, the mattress propped up, resting his head on his favorite pillow, which I'd brought from home, blue sky and leafy green trees the motif of the linen. He looked pale and tired, had a white plastic bracelet around his wrist, wearing a tank top and his slinky silver jogging shorts. That was the best I could come up with for a hospital ensemble, his jogging clothes. Steve never wore pajamas, never wore underwear, had only one pair of raggedy briefs saved for doctor's appointments. He had a drawer full of the same white socks, and each morning he'd fish two from the jumble. I'd always liked the pragmatism of this system, and admired his refusal of underwear altogether, a small private rebellion.

"How many tumors are there?" I asked the doctor.

"There are several," he said.

"Where are they?" I asked. I needed to visualize the layout of the aggressor, like playing Battleship when I was a kid. Players who guessed the exact position of their opponent's ships won.

"Lumbars two, three, four." Dr. Demmons faced Steve as he spoke, ignoring me.

"Well, what can you do? What's the prognosis?" I said.

The doctor glared at me and turned back to Steve.

"I want her here," Steve said to the doctor, firmly.

Dr. Demmons sighed. "There's really nothing we can do. Some radiation along the spine might help with the pain."

"What about chemotherapy?" I asked.

"We could try a few sessions of chemotherapy," Dr. Demmons said to Steve, "but you'd just get sick and weak. It might not prolong your life. It might even shorten it." It seemed that he hadn't even considered a plan for Steve.

"What are we supposed to do?" I asked.

"I suggest you go home," he said, wanting to be rid of us both, it was clear. In spite of his training at the famed Mayo Clinic, which he mentioned often, Dr. Demmons was helpless, his years of schooling, his knowledge and experience, in Steve's case, all for naught.

"How long does he have to live?" I asked. Steve could not articulate these questions, could not say, "how long do *I* have to live?" Speaking of him in third person as if he were a stranger in our room, a nameless *he*, semantically at least, we could hold his fate at bay.

"We don't like to guess," the doctor said.

"You must have some idea," I insisted.

"I'd say anywhere from two weeks to two months." Dr. Demmons must have noticed the shock on our faces. "Six months at the outside," he added, "but I'd be surprised."

The doctor walked out, leaving us in the room with his forecast: the trajectory of Steve's life—which statistically should be another forty-seven years—was now two months.

I'm sure I wept; I've been a weeper all my life, but I can't recall. You would imagine that the memory of those hours would singe deeply into my psyche, that I would memorize them as a film clip. But memory gets muddled at such news; the mind ceases to function as its highest cognitive levels: reasoning, judgment, abstract thought. My mind, benumbed, could make no sense of that.

The next day, Dr. Demmons and Dr. Lin spoke with Steve's parents. Afterward, Bill and Louise and I stood in a small examining room down the hall, hugging and crying. "I guess we should put him in a hospice," Louise said, dabbing her eyes.

"No way," I said. Steve and I both were appalled at his mother's suggestion, that she was ready to accept Steve's fate as God's will, her only son, her first born, the beautiful white-haired boy with big blue eyes, for whom strangers stopped on the street to exclaim how pretty. I'd seen his baby pictures; Steve was a sweet-faced child, a handsome teenager, a fair and beautiful young man. When he and I walked down the street or into a restaurant, it was Steve who turned heads. In the hospital now, though, I saw already the xylophone of ribs under his skin, new hollows in his cheeks.

But hospice? Another course I'd taken in college was Death and Dying: Loss as a Part of Life, a sociology class in which we'd read Kübler-Ross. (If I weren't a skeptic, I might believe that my course selections, Microbiology of Cancer, and Death and Dying, weren't random, but karmic preparation for what I'd encounter.)

Over the next week, Steve was wheeled out of his room for radiation treatments on his vertebrae just above the tailbone, where the pain was most acute. There were tiny blue Xs tattooed on his spine like on a treasure map. Once it was confirmed that Steve had tumors, I began to notice suspicious bumps under *my* skin, near my eyelid, my palm. My mother assured me that these were harmless fatty deposits, calcium build ups, bone spurs. Still, I worried. If cancer could spring up seemingly overnight in Steve, who was robustly strong and virile, then how could I know what was going on inside my body? Bodies could not be trusted anymore.

In college I had worked nights in the library at the University of Massachusetts nearly full-time. I was the slowest shelver, taking a few minutes to read a bit of each book before placing it in its rightful, decimally-ordained place. I learned to navigate the labyrinthine, chokingly-overheated library. Reference was my basilica. Here I bowed: the reference librarians, my deities. For a while, I thought of earning a Master's in Library Science, joining the ranks of the keepers of knowledge. In reference, the world is catalogued. If one can locate the almost esoteric codes that are key to the system, if one can decipher the indices, one can know everything. Libraries housed answers; that's what I believed.

Each afternoon while Steve was in St. Joe's, I drove to the University of Michigan library to research cancer treatments. Phyllis's company sold most of her products during the holidays, so February was slow. Since I was paid by the hour, she didn't mind my short days. I read about Linus Pauling's experiments with Vitamin C, an antioxidant that inhibits cancer cells, which feed on oxygen. I bought high-milligram, timed-released vitamin C for Steve. One morning on his rounds, Dr. Demmons offhandedly picked up the bottle of vitamin C from Steve's night stand.

"What's this?" he said.

"Vitamin C," Steve replied. "It's supposed to fight cancer."

"Ha!" the doctor said.

I glowered. "Linus Pauling won a Nobel prize," I said, unaware that Pauling's Nobel was not for his claims about Vitamin C and cancer, for which he was scorned by the scientific community.

"It might help if you have a cold," Dr. Demmons said.

Nevertheless, Steve asked Dr. Demmons to order vitamins for him, and thereafter a Flintstones chewable multivitamin appeared on his lunch tray each day, a yellow Barney or pink Fred, violet Wilma.

A day later, I asked Dr. Demmons if he knew of any experimental treatments. "No. There aren't any programs," he assured me. But when I called around the hospitals in Detroit, I found experimental protocols at Henry Ford and Harper Hospital and Wayne State. Through cancer hotlines, I turned up experimental programs across the country. The Ford and Harper's programs had long waiting lists, or Steve was not eligible due to his type of cancer and its advanced stage. Some of the experimental regimens didn't sound promising, or the side effects seemed too severe.

Beyond the auspices of the mainstream medical community, there were dozens of alternative treatments, all denounced by the American Cancer Society. Every day Steve and I considered a new plan for his treatment. One day, we decided that the laetrile clinics in Mexico were the best option, and I gathered costs on flights, researched travel visas. I called my family to tell them we were leaving for Tijuana. The next day I found another treatment that sounded more promising and suddenly we'd decided to head for the Bahamas for complete blood transfusion therapy at a cost of $10,000 per session—Steve's house money, his stash from working overtime, kept in our bedroom closet in a small fireproof box.

Two days before Steve and I planned on leaving for the Bahamas, I found an article in the library written by a doctor who'd had cancer. The doctor argued that the alternative treatments (specifically the Bahamas clinic) were a hoax. He argued that if something worked, the medical establishment wouldn't deny it to patients. What would be their motive? Doctors got cancer, so did their spouses and children. There was no malign medical cabal withholding treatment from cancer patients. But there were plenty of unproven programs, the proprietors of which were happy to take the last savings of desperate people. The treatments often caused patients to die sooner than they might have, and far away from family and friends in some foreign country, in a city like Tijuana.

I'd been to Tijuana when Sally and I drove cross country after I graduated high school. I pictured the dusty dirt roads of Tijuana, the shacks just off the main street, collages of corrugated tin, scrap lumber, and cardboard, the barefoot children yanking on my shirt, hawking packs of gum. The article swayed me with its logic, though I was tempted to hide it from Steve. I didn't want to be Cassandra, bearer of bad news, deflator of hope, but ultimately it was his decision. I sat on the end of the bed while Steve read the article, watched his brow furrow, watched his expression fall away as he finished reading.

We cancelled the trip to the clinic in the Bahamas. We were disheartened, but not resigned. There was still reason for hope. In a medical journal, I'd uncovered an actuarial table for cancer survival rates. A column along the side of the chart listed varieties of the disease, including *adenocarcinoma*. Across the top row I located "stage IV," and where my fingers met on the page was the figure .00001. This statistic felt like an opening, a small rent in a high concrete wall. The doctors had said with certainty that there was *nothing* anyone could do for Steve, that his case was *terminal*. But my chart refuted that. My chart proved that someone with fourth stage adenocarcinoma had survived, some *one* person beat the odds, some extraordinary, singularly determined person somewhere in the world, and I could visualize that one person among 100,000: Steve.

"Steve," I said, "tell yourself each day you are going to get better and better."

"I'm going to get better and better," Steve replied, slightly loopy from painkillers. "I'll be the best."

One night Steve's chiropractor, Dr. Epstein, stopped by with a brochure from American International Hospital in Zion, Illinois, which offered a holistic approach to cancer—traditional treatment combined with alternative and experimental procedures. This sounded perfect to us, the comfort of traditional medicine, the hope of new methods, a perspective that treated mind *and* body, heart and soul. Steve called AIH the next day and spoke with Dr. Ranulfo Sanchez.

"What did he say?" I asked Steve after he hung up.

"He says to get there as fast as I can."

I booked two tickets to Chicago, and arranged to rent a car.

Steve's parents were anxious. "All the doctors are Filipino," his mother said, thumbing through the brochure.

"They have good medical schools in the Philippines," I replied, though I didn't know that, knew little about the Philippines, couldn't have located the islands on a map. "It's better than a hospice," I said.

That afternoon, Steve told Dr. Demmons that he was transferring. The doctor shook his head, and left the room. Until then, Dr. Demmons had domain over Steve, withholding and releasing information as he saw fit, determining the course of treatment and quality of life, offering Steve a nominal choice (painful and ravishing chemotherapy or sent home to die). But Steve withdrew, which rendered the doctor powerless. He took his body somewhere else.

10. Body Snatchers

Youth is fertile soil in which hope blossoms. Sometimes ignorance, naiveté are our best assets. Ignorance, fueled by sheer will, allowed Steve and me to charge headlong into the unknown. The morning after Steve spoke with Dr. Sanchez at AIH, he checked out of St. Joe's and we boarded a plane for Chicago, zooming through the air at 500 miles per hour. Given his prognosis, we had no time to waste. Perhaps, too, we did not want the time to ponder our decision, to let doubt pry its way between hope and possibility.

On the plane, I pulled Steve's medical reports from the manila envelope. I recognized Latin roots of words: sternum, femur, cranium. Dr. Demmons hadn't mentioned that, along with the tumors along Steve's spine, there were tumors on his breastbone, thigh, skull, hip. *Widespread.* The report was disturbing, as was Dr. Lin's final note in Steve's chart: *It is very sad to see that the patient cannot accept the poor prognosis.* I pushed the forms back into the envelope, didn't mention anything to Steve who was staring out the window at clouds and sky. This was his first plane ride.

At O'Hare, the Hertz agent refused to rent me the car I'd reserved.

"The person on the phone didn't tell me I needed a credit card," I said with strained politeness. The clerk shrugged. I didn't own a credit card, neither did Steve. I'd brought cash to pay for a week, and an extra $200 for the deposit, which cleaned out my checking account. "I am with a very ill man in great pain." I pointed to Steve slumped in a plastic chair nearby. "We need to get to the hospital an hour away."

The clerk called the manager, who agreed to phone my employer. Luckily, Maggie, who worked part-time, was still packing boxes. She verified my employment, and the clerk handed me the keys. "We're on our way now," I said to Steve, but first we had to board a shuttle to the rental car lot, though the salesperson on the phone had promised delivery of our car to the terminal. My efforts to minimize Steve's discomfort, to take care of everything, were failing. Steve's pain medication was wearing off. (Since he was no longer under their care, the doctors at St. Joseph's would not write a prescription for pain medication. That morning, they'd given Steve two morphine tablets, an eight hour dose.)

Steve reclined in the passenger seat of the car and in the dusk I drove north along the shoreline of Lake Michigan. Fifty minutes later, following directions from the hospital receptionist, we arrived at a single-story, L-shaped brick building. It was dark and cold, late February. The lights in the building were off; all the doors were locked. The place was closed. This was the moment I began to panic. No pain killers, six hours by car away from our apartment, just Steve and me, neither of us too worldly, neither of us thirty yet. Steve waited in the car while I walked around the building, crunching through snow and trampling shrubbery, peering in the windows like a peeping Tom. I saw a man and rapped on the window.

"Are you open?" I shouted.

He shook his head.

"But we called! They're expecting us." I was really going to cry now.

"This is the clinic," the man yelled through the window. "You could try the hospital around the corner." He gave me muffled directions.

Five minutes later, Steve and I checked into American International Hospital, a four-story, seventy-bed facility. Steve's room had four single beds; three were vacant. The bedspreads were threadbare, with small moth-eaten holes, which alarmed me. What kind of shabby, fly-by-night place had we come to, leaving behind the gleaming 600-bed St. Joseph's in Ypsilanti, where Steve'd had his own private room? It was

8:00 p.m., and the nurse on duty, a pretty Filipina named Fay ordered us each a tray of food, and sat on the end of Steve's bed chatting with us while we ate.

The food was good: brown rice, and freshly squeezed carrot-celery juice, a bowl of fresh fruit (not soggy canned chunks like at St. Joe's). I felt reassured. I told Fay about mistaking the clinic for the hospital and we all laughed, though an hour earlier I'd been close to tears. This was the motif of our life suddenly, polar opposites: good and evil doctors, life and death decisions, broken up then back together—a tacit understanding now between Steve and me, love a stronger bond than the formalities of partnership: cohabitation, legal status, terms of endearment: boyfriend, girlfriend. That night, the nurses let me sleep in the empty bed next to Steve.

In the morning Steve's doctors introduced themselves. Dr. Sanchez was a handsome, square-jawed Filipino, stout and sturdy-framed with a broad intelligent face. His colleague, Dr. Melijor, was a quiet, slight man, also Filipino. Steve recited Dr. Demmons' prognosis.

"We don't give up so easily," Dr. Sanchez said. He was our instant hero, our savior. "Want to see your x-rays?" he asked Steve, and invited me along.

In his office, the doctor clipped Steve's nuclear scans to a light panel mounted on the wall. Steve's skeleton glowed against the gray film, a grisaille of his body. Small black dots were sprayed from his skull to his kneecaps, as if someone had plugged him with bird shot. Thoracic vertebrae, ilium, sacrum. It was a frightening lesson in anatomy. Dr. Sanchez seemed unfazed by these results, but I was shocked by the numerous black dots, far more than I'd envisioned when Dr. Demmons back in Ypsilanti spoke vaguely of "multiple tumors." "Multiple" meant six or seven, a sixpack, a touchdown, a number we could beat. I counted more than two dozen specks on the little x-ray man that was Steve.

Not to mention his liver, marbleized, like a high-priced cut of beef, with cancer. I'd envisioned the liver tumor as an appendage on the organ, a big polyp like the puffball mushrooms that pop up after a rain: white, the size of a golf ball, easily cut away. Instead the cancer cells had mingled throughout Steve's liver like the aliens in *The Body Snatchers*. Though shocking at first, the scans demystified Steve's condition. The x-rays made Steve's cancer tangible in a way it wasn't when the disease was hidden under skin. The enigma of illness was removed; disease was reduced to biology. Cancer, in aggregate, was only the sum of its parts—black spots on the screen. Now we had to begin erasing those spots.

That afternoon, Dr. Sanchez surgically implanted an Infusaport in Steve's chest, a catheter into his subclavian vein, the largest in the body, a direct line to the heart. The Infusaport prevented the toxic chemicals from burning the skin at the typical infusion site, the wrist. The port of the catheter, a clear plastic tube slightly less round in circumference than a drinking straw, hung an inch or so outside Steve's skin, just below his collar bone. When not in use, the port was covered with gauze and bandages. Twice daily, a nurse flushed the tube with heparin, an anticoagulant that prevented blood clots from forming, which could break loose, travel the vein, and cause a heart attack.

While Steve was in surgery, I perused the hospital bulletin board and noticed a room for rent, ten dollars a night. I called a woman named Noma, who gave me directions to her house and promised to leave the porch lit. Then I called Phyllis, my boss. I'd left her a note saying I was terribly sorry, but I had to take an immediate leave of absence for an indeterminate amount of time, and that I'd understand if she needed to replace me. She knew Steve's prognosis, so I assumed she'd accept my decision, but I was nervous as I stood at the pay phone in the hallway of the hospital.

"How could you leave me in the lurch like this?" Phyllis said. "What am I going to do for the convention next week?"

I was supposed to represent Phyllis's business in her booth at a trade convention in Detroit. "It wasn't very responsible of you to go running off without any notice. This is the worst possible time."

I could barely speak. I wanted to remind her that $5.50 an hour with no benefits bought some of my time, some of my labor, but not my loyalty. I did not say this, though; it would have been rude. I was raised with manners: even in the face of heartlessness, be polite to your boss.

"I'm sorry," I said. "I think you would have done the same thing. Can't you find somebody else?" People walking by in the hallway stared at me.

"When will you be back?" she asked.

"I really can't say at this point, but I'll let you know."

The thought that I would actually return to work hadn't occurred to me. Steve and I had moved into a state of immediacy, dealing with life a minute at a time. Raising our eyes to the future—even a week ahead—was not an option.

Visitation officially ended at eight p.m., but the nurses understood that hours mattered and allowed me to stay until eleven. Then I walked to a small ranch house three blocks away. The couple who owned the house, Noma and Emil, were up when I arrived.

"Wipe down the shower before you get out. Don't use too much toilet paper. And use the towel more than once," Noma said, scolding, like she knew I'd transgress. She was a tiny woman with a pile of messy gray hair, and one sharp, pointy tooth protruding from her mouth, like an egg tooth a baby bird uses to peck its way out of a shell.

"Who've you got in the hospital?" she asked.

"My boyfriend."

"He got cancer?" She didn't wait for an answer. "People come from all over to go to that hospital. We've had people from Florida, Kentucky, California. We got another room we rent besides yours."

"Tell her about the one from New Zealand!" Emil added. "He stayed right in the room you're staying in," he said, as if I were privileged. "Stayed here twice. His wife had cancer. She died." Emil had filmy blue eyes and hair that was sugar-white with bangs cut straight across his forehead. He looked like an old angel.

"Emil and I are blessed with good health, thank the lord," Noma said. "Emil broke his ankle forty years ago. It was healed by a miracle at our church and it never bothered him since, right Em?"

"I'm eighty-four years old and still march with the Brothers of Zion band." Emil opened a closet and pulled out a red wool coat and matching pants with gold braiding up the seams. "It's no coincidence you're in Zion," he said. "This is a holy town. Miracles take place all the time."

Emil described their church, the crutches and prosthetics mounted on its walls from people who'd cast them away after being healed. His story tracked with history. In 1901, John Alexander Dowie, a faith healer, founded Zion as a "City of God." The entire town was built by 5,000 devotees who volunteered their labor. For much of the early 1900s people migrated to Zion in search of salvation and miracles, healing through divine intervention. Dowie had even banned doctors within the city limits.

Steve and I had not traveled to Zion for a miracle from the church, but a scientific cure, the doctors modern day clerics. Besides, with its Kentucky Fried Chicken and McDonald's, boarded-up buildings and seedy streets, Zion didn't look like any kind of holy place, just a down-on-its-luck town along the flat, pebbly shore of Lake Michigan, an hour north of Chicago and twenty minutes south of Wisconsin.

The next morning, when I told Steve about Noma and Emil, he said, "You're too polite. You should have just said, 'I'm tired and I'm going to bed.'" His words seemed so simple, like abracadabra, but I couldn't conjure them the night before. Steve walked into the bathroom and I trailed him. I hated to let him out of my sight. When he pulled down his jogging shorts, I noticed that his body had changed. He had roundish hips and puffy curves like a woman. His legs were swollen. His skin was jiggly and loose. I poked the bloated flesh as if I could pop it. It was terribly disconcerting, this morphing of Steve's body, this shape-shifting into a different form overnight. Steve couldn't see the change as there was no full-length mirror, but when he stepped on the scale, he'd gained eleven pounds.

Edema, Fay told us, water retention caused by the new pain medication. Dr. Sanchez switched Steve back to morphine and Dilaudid, which he'd started at St. Joseph's. The morphine pills were tiny, round, and bright purple; they reminded me of power pills that Underdog, that cartoon character from my childhood, kept in a secret-cache ring. Morphine is long-acting but didn't alleviate the worst of Steve's pain, so for acute relief, he took Dilaudid, squarish, pale-yellow pills that looked like babies' first teeth.

After the first night, Noma and Emil didn't bother to leave the porch lit. I'd arrive there around midnight and read for a while before turning off the lamp. On my third night there, I was poked awake by noises in the kitchen: a spoon clinking against a dish; footsteps; cupboards opening and shutting; a toilet flushing. The sequence of noises repeated, seemed to be a cycle: spoon, steps, cupboard, flush. Again.

I heard snoring from Noma and Emil's room. They would have had to pass my room to get to the kitchen, but I hadn't heard anyone in the hall. I became convinced there was a ghost just outside my door, a tortured soul who refused to accept death and was stuck for eternity in his last moment of life, compelled to make his final meal again and again. I pulled my blankets to my chin though I was sweating. My heart pounded, pushing my tired blood, echoing in the small room. I prayed. *Please God, don't let it come in here.* I lay stiff with fear until the gray light of dawn when spirits are banished until finally, from exhaustion, I fell asleep.

I woke mid-morning, groggy. Emil's white toupee was fitted on a Styrofoam head on the kitchen table, his teeth in a tumbler of water on the bathroom sink. I closed my eyes while I brushed my teeth so I didn't have to stare at the dentures. I asked Noma if she'd heard noises in the night.

"Just me eating my cereal," she said. "I get up about three every morning and have some cereal."

"What about the flushing?" I asked.

"That's the pump clearing water out of the basement."

In the daytime, I could get along. There were people, objects, events to hold on to, give texture to time, divide up space. But at night, alone and in the dark, I could lose my way, lose my mind.

It was ten when I arrived at the hospital and climbed in bed with Steve, as if I were joining him in his body, unzipping his skin like it was a space suit, and snuggling in. By then, Steve had two roommates, Greg and Chuck. Greg was olive-complected, medium-built. He owned his own pest extermination business in South Carolina. I hypothesized that the poisons he'd sprayed for years to kill cockroaches and termites had seeped into his body and perhaps had caused his cancer. When I asked, he said, "I don't think it's related."

Since Steve and I had learned of his cancer, we blamed everything and everyone according to whatever I uncovered in my research. When we found out that charred food was carcinogenic, we blamed ourselves for grilling out so often, all winter long on the veranda of our apartment. We blamed Steve's vocation as an electrician when I read that exposure to high tension electrical wires increased the incidence of cancer. We blamed the stress of Steve's life: his divorce, our breakup. I'd found a chart that measured stress by assigning numerical values to life events. Death of a spouse, divorce, job loss, and relocation topped the list. When we totaled Steve's points for the last two years of his life, he was in the highest category for illness and accidents. There were no points for happy events—like falling in love—that might cancel or mitigate the stress.

We pointed the finger at everything, but specifically at nothing. Even the doctors couldn't say why Steve had cancer, or where, definitively, it had originated (pancreas, liver, bile duct?). But Steve and I continued to blame, trying to find a logic to this situation, some reasonable explanation for why a healthy young man should be dying so swiftly.

Greg was young too, twenty-seven. Nearly all day Greg slept or read his Bible. He rarely spoke, but frequently groaned or vomited or buzzed for the nurses. Hand him his urine jug (which was at the foot of his bed), fix his pillow, bring him a drink, as if he were at a resort.

"Quit your sniveling," Steve taunted. "Get out of bed."

Greg smiled. He seemed to like Steve's chiding. "You're lucky to have Maureen here," Greg said, as if I were not standing right there.

I was taken aback: Steve was not lucky, I thought. There was no way that anyone could consider Steve a lucky man, unless of course they were speaking of bad luck. But it was considerate of Greg to mention me. Few patients had the luxury of being accompanied to the hospital by a loved one. Because I was young, because I didn't have children to care for, or an important job that would be difficult to leave behind, a big mortgage to pay, or any kind of business to run, I had nothing to lose traveling to Zion. Then again, I had everything to lose: Steve.

Chuck, Steve's other roommate, was a fiftyish executive who'd quit smoking ten years earlier, but developed lung cancer anyway. Chuck languished in his bed four feet from Steve, privacy afforded via a thin curtain suspended from a ceiling track, which the nurses pulled when they drained the mucus from Chuck's lungs. Steve and I couldn't see that procedure, but we heard it (a rasping, liquidy noise, like when Nate or Lisa sucked the last drops of soda through a straw). When it was over, we spied the glass receptacle filled with greenish, yellowy-white matter.

Steve kept his curtain open so he could see out the windows beyond Chuck's bed, but Chuck was not easy to look at. He had a clear tube taped to his cheek and inserted into his nostril. Oxygen from tanks on the side of his bed flowed continuously through the tube into his drowning, malignant lungs, all day and night. Chuck was an earth bound scuba diver. He breathed loud and heavy, and coughed wet phlegmy coughs which temporarily paralyzed his wife Sheila's kinetic fingers as she sat in a chair by his bed knitting violently, as if she were weaving Chuck a new set of lungs.

In the afternoons, Steve and I walked around the hallways exploring the hospital, or sat in the sun room at the end of the hall, which overlooked a duck pond across the street. We visited the tiny dark chapel with its one pew and miniature carpeted altar, so small it was like our own private church, no bigger than a bathroom. We walked through the cafeteria where visitors could purchase the same choice of fresh-squeezed juices served to patients, carrot-celery, parsley-radish-tomato, a dozen other combinations, and healthy meals like lentil-loaf and tofu. American International Hospital's beds were mostly occupied by cancer patients. The patients who didn't have cancer were treated mainly for foot problems. Cancer and bunions, their two specialties. I wished Steve was on the bunion ward.

Steve held his I.V. pole like a staff, rolling it along the linoleum on its wheeled base. Glass containers and clear plastic bags hung from the pole, one with clear liquid minerals to fortify Steve's body, the other with liquid vitamins. Three small bottles—six ouncers, like stubby baby bottles—were chemicals: 5-FU, adriamycin, mitomycin. The names reminded me of the defoliants that were dropped in Vietnam to denude jungles. These chemicals zapped cells that reproduced rapidly, like cancer cells, like hair cells, like cells that line the stomach and mouth. All these liquids fed into the catheter in Steve's chest, flowing into the big subclavian vein, direct to Steve's heart like a fast underground train.

This was decelerated, or "fractured dose" chemotherapy, though, administered over a five day period. At St. Joe's in Ypsilanti, the chemicals would have been dispensed in a matter of hours, like an illegal nighttime dumping of toxic waste.

Days in the hospital passed slowly. Flowers arrived from Steve's parents, with a card: *When God closes a door, he opens a window.* I arranged the card and bouquet on the night stand, opened the curtains and watched activity below, cars and people. Fat, slow winter flies buzzed against the sealed glass. They appeared out of nowhere it seemed. Steve was more social than I, so he popped his head into any inhabited room and chatted with patients. We were lucky to find American International Hospital early, Steve learned from his rounds. He heard horror stories about the traditional chemotherapy regimens that beat up the body, like muggers, the patient left nearly dead, or the alternative cures, some that we'd considered just a week before, the small fortunes people lost while they sickened.

Steve befriended the women in the room across the hall, Ramona and Sue and Estherine; there were far more women on the cancer unit than men. Ramona and Sue had breast cancer; Estherine had cancer of the uterus. They were young, these women, none over forty-five, though they all looked older in their obvious wigs with too shiny, too bouncy hair, or bald scalps with fluffy stray wisps. Steve favored Georgia from down the hall, refined and genteel in her elegant robe, a turban framing her high cheekbones, deep set eyes, gently aquiline nose. Georgia never joined the camaraderie of the other women, playing cards or board games, ordering out for pizza as if they were at a sleepover or summer camp.

A social worker visited Steve and invited him to a support group, and a psychologist explained the counseling service, how it was important to deal with the emotional and psychological aspects of illness, to treat the disease holistically. Mind over body, mind connected to body. A physical therapist discussed pain management with us, and offered Steve a TENS unit (transcutaneous electrical nerve stimulation), a gadget the size of a small transistor radio, which dispensed low-level charges. For years Steve worked as an electrician, careful to avoid dangerous currents, yet now these volts could provide relief from pain. Steve and I were buoyed by the attention, the all-out effort to save him, as if he were important, as if he were savable.

Fay prepared me for taking care of Steve at home. She taught me to clean the catheter in Steve's chest: to swab the tender pink incision with alcohol; apply antiseptic ointment with a Q-tip; fill a syringe with heparin, which was packaged in miniature single-dose bottles, one-inch tall. She watched me tap the syringe to release bubbles so that I didn't inject air into Steve's veins and kill him that way. I pushed the plunger into the port in Steve's chest slowly (he could feel a rapid injection), then replaced the dressing.

On the tenth day in Zion, after twenty-four days of hospitalization (including the two weeks at St. Joseph's), Steve was discharged with orders to return in three weeks. I'd returned the rental car after our arrival to save money, and so we were transported back to O'Hare in the hospital's aging limousine: black, funereal, donated, but luxuriously comfortable. On the highway, people passing in cars stared into our opaque windows. Like spirits, we could see them but they couldn't see us. They must have thought that Steve and I were rich and lucky, mistakenly envying us in our private, fancy car. It was mildly satisfying to feel privileged, even if untrue.

Steve and I gazed out the windows at the scenery rushing by, miles and miles of silvery farm fields still dormant in late winter. It was hypnotic. Abruptly though, buildings and pavement and civilization appeared as we approached the airport. Passing through this convergence of landscapes, we spotted a deer behind a chain link fence along the highway. How strange, I thought, this feral creature so close to the city, how lost it must be, how frightened.

11. Forget-me-nots

The day before I'd left for Europe, just two months after meeting Steve in New York, I cut a curl of my hair and presented it to him in a cardboard match box, a piece of myself, which he kept with his other treasures—boy scout badges, arrowheads, fossils—in an antique wooden chest on his dresser, as if the lock of hair was a talisman, able to ward off enemies, like the hair of Medusa, which Steve sometimes called me. Within a day of arriving home from Zion, Steve awoke to find hair on his pillow, whole chunks like the curl I'd given him. Hair loss is a physically painless aspect of chemotherapy; you cannot feel the shedding, but it's the most conspicuous, and in some ways the most troubling. We knew that this loss, the death of these cells, was not caused by the disease but by its remedy.

I continued my research on holistic healing, nearly memorizing Earl Mindell's *Vitamin Bible*, the only bible I consulted. Unlike Steve's mother, I placed my faith in science. I determined a regimen for Steve, arranging vitamins in an empty egg carton, a handful each day, plus spoonfuls of Vitamin C powder mixed with juice. The recommended daily allowance for Vitamin C is less than half a gram, but Steve and I gradually increased our dose to eleven grams. (Linus Pauling, who took thirty grams a day, claimed vitamin C could extend a life span by twenty-five years. He died at 93, four years short of his calculation, after a long bout with cancer.)

Vitamin A is reputed to fight cancer, but it's toxic if ingested in high levels. The body transforms beta-carotene into vitamin A without harm, nature's own alchemy. Carrots are rich in beta-carotene, so I bought a centrifugal juicer to extract carrot juice. Steve could drink as much carrot juice as he wanted with the only side effect being the ruddling of his complexion. Each morning I scrubbed two pounds of organic carrots to fill one tall glass of cold, sweet juice for Steve, and repeated the process at night.

Fish liver oil was thought to inhibit cancer, but in 1986 it wasn't common to find fish oil pills in health food stores. So instead I bought empty gelatin caps and a bottle of cod liver oil, and using one of Steve's syringes for the heparin I injected into his catheter, I attempted to fill the tiny capsules, coating them and myself with the rank, slimy oil. For days my hands reeked of rotten fish.

I met with Phyllis, my boss. She'd already hired a new administrative assistant, Kristin. Phyllis asked me to train Kristin, and I proposed to Phyllis that she keep me on twenty hours a week to take care of public relations and marketing. She agreed, and allowed me time off to accompany Steve on future trips to Zion. I was grateful for her flexibility.

One afternoon as I was explaining a procedure to Kristin, she stood abruptly. "Just slow down!" she said. "For three days you've been spewing extraneous bullshit!" I struggled to maintain composure. Since Steve had been diagnosed, a reservoir of hot tears swelled just under the surface of my skin, like Steve's edema, a vast subcutaneous aquifer. "Kristin, I'm leaving again next week and I won't be around to answer questions." Maggie, who'd been quietly taping cartons, offered a look of sympathy. I attempted to speak slower, to sift the information for Kristin, but I had trouble breathing and found myself accelerating to accommodate my shallow breaths.

The next day Kristin apologized. She did not think she'd have as much responsibility with a measly seven-dollar-per-hour job. Seven dollars per hour? When I learned that Kristin was earning more than me, I went to speak with Phyllis in her office upstairs. "I have a year experience on this job. How can you expect me to train a replacement who is getting paid more than me?"

"I think you're taking advantage of your situation," Phyllis said. "I can't believe you'd play on my pity."

"This has nothing to do with Steve," I said. "It's just not fair."

Phyllis's accusation shocked me. I couldn't possibly have been as calculating as she claimed. I was operating in the mode of raw reaction; this was purely a business matter. But maybe my reaction was overblown. Against the scrim of Steve's life, the unfairness of his fate, this small injustice was magnified.

Alone all afternoon, Steve worked on stained glass projects. We'd started lessons together the year before, but I lacked the patience for the craft, which Steve had mastered quickly. In his workshop, a tiny second bedroom in our apartment, he was surrounded by glass: large panels with swirling colors; acid-etched patterns; rough textures; expensive milky opalescent glass; and boxes and boxes of scraps. My favorite glass was the clear, wafer thin, hand-blown sheets with small air bubbles trapped inside that looked like raindrops. When balanced against a window pane, that glass turned any day into a rainy day.

Steve kept a box of wildflowers he'd picked in a field near our apartment: Queen Anne's lace and tiny forget-me-nots, orange hawkweed, lavender Johnny-jump-ups and blue toadflax. He pressed the blossoms between two boards until they were dry and completely flat, like torn bits of parchment. Then he arranged petals and leaves and small feathers he'd found—plumes from the breasts of wild pheasants, which shimmered like moiré in the light—and butterfly wings. Steve had a collection of butterflies he'd found dead on the ground, uncrushed but frozen, as if the air itself had killed them. All these pieces and parts and shapes and colors he suspended between two pieces of glass, a tiny still-life garden that bloomed forever.

Aside from the efforts to heal Steve's body, there was his attitude to alter. I read a book by the Simontons, a husband and wife team, who believed that people could help to heal themselves through visualization and positive thinking. Each night in bed, Steve ran a filmstrip in his mind, white blood cells squashing cancer cells like June bugs on a leaf. I gave Steve a card offering another scene to visualize: *Keep thinking about our home in the country, with a garden and a stream and nature surrounding us. This is going to happen. We'll make it happen.* I believed in sheer willpower, the lesson of my upbringing, that anything could be accomplished with "elbow-grease," as my mother called it—my mother, finisher of rooms, builder of a half-way-in-ground pool in our backyard.

Convinced that Steve needed to see a counselor, I called an ad from the back of Ann Arbor's alternative paper, which read, "Life Cycle Counseling: Illness, Death, Divorce, Job Loss," and spoke to Cendra Lynn, Ph.D. "We want someone who believes in the Simonton's method," I said. I didn't want anyone telling me that Steve couldn't heal himself. This seemed crucial. Dr. Demmons at St. Joe's offered no hope. Dr. Sanchez in Zion offered a slim margin, but the odds were not in Steve's favor. Without any enduring faith in God and a waning confidence in traditional medicine, who was left to do the job of healing Steve? He and I. It made sense, this ability to save ourselves, to control our biology with the brain. Of course the mind could rule the dumb ox of the body.

"I'm familiar with their theories," Cendra said. I could detect hesitance in her voice. "Why don't you come in and we can talk?"

"I have to convince Steve to make an appointment," I confessed.

"What about you?" she asked. This question seemed odd. I was not the one who was ill. I was perfectly healthy and completely in control, not only of my situation, but Steve's.

"Let's make an appointment anyway," she said, "and we'll see what we can do about Steve." Cendra's voice was gentle, convincing, but there was a hitch.

"I don't have any insurance," I said. "How much do you charge?"

"Let's not worry about that," she said. I appreciated her use of the inclusive pronoun, *us*, as if she'd joined the fight already. "I have a sliding fee scale. I'm sure I can accommodate you."

When I suggested counseling to Steve— as I had earlier in our relationship when we were fighting—he wasn't willing. "You go," he said, "and tell me about it."

Cendra's office was in an old Victorian in a quiet residential neighborhood in Ann Arbor. The building was in need of a paint job, but daffodils bloomed in small plots in the front yard, and the waiting room was sunny and pleasant. Cendra wore a colorful muu muu, her breasts swinging loosely beneath. She propped her bare feet on an ottoman in her office, tossed back her frizzy auburn hair. She had pretty blue eyes, downturned at the corners as if she automatically sympathized with me. Fair and freckled, Irish looking, with a high forehead and narrow face, she looked to be in her late thirties.

I began by talking about the Simonton's ideas, how Steve could heal himself.

"If Steve's mind has the power to cure illness, does that mean he could have created it?" Cendra asked.

"He's had a lot of anger and stress," I said, "so maybe." My attitude was as old as medicine itself. In 200 A.D., Galen observed that "melancholy" women were more likely to get breast cancer than "sanguine" women. Galen, the "father of medicine," was perhaps the first to blame the victim.

"Why would anyone give himself a horrible disease like cancer?" Cendra asked me. "Does that mean if he doesn't heal himself, then he doesn't want to be healed?"

I didn't have answers to Cendra's questions.

"Cancer is a biological disease," she said quietly. "You can't help getting cancer any more than coming down with the flu."

I felt guilty holding Steve responsible for his disease and its cure both. It wasn't a fair expectation. After all, when I suffered a simple cold, I was a whiny baby. I couldn't will away my sinus headaches induced by Michigan's muggy summer air, so how could I expect Steve to vanquish cancer with mental fortitude? Half-way through the session, I gave up on the Simontons. How easily I changed my mind, it seemed. But there were so many different theories, and I couldn't tease apart rational ideas from pure desire. I *needed* for there to be a way for Steve and me, who'd dreamed of self-sufficiency, to cure him. What seems like unchecked hubris—that I could be elemental in saving Steve, where doctors had failed!—was denial of Steve's disturbing prognosis. Denial, the psyche's own morphine, is refusal; refusal is an exercise of power.

"Let's make another appointment," Cendra said. "This one for you. Don't worry about Steve. He'll come if he wants to."

Her words jolted me: *Don't worry about Steve.* That's all I'd been doing for two months. Cendra gave me permission to draw myself into the picture, the frame that had been occupied solely by Steve. When she offered to charge me a quarter of her normal fee, I realized that she was some kind of fairy godmother. "I knew we would click," she said as I left. "We have the same hair."

At home, after Steve regained some strength, we tried to resume our normal life, but resuming our normal life would have meant that I'd live with Sally, and that Steve and I would be separating. There was no returning to that status, not when Steve needed me.

On a Friday night, we dined at Luthauser's, Saline's only fancy restaurant, but Steve was restless and uncomfortable in the high-backed wooden chairs, and impatient with the waitress who seemed to take such a long time. He was self-conscious, believing that people were staring at him with his bald head and wan face (they were). Steve was thin, the degree of skinny that people equate with illness. His jeans sagged, and I could see his pelvis and the knob of tailbone. So after that evening, we stayed home mostly. At night we watched television or rented movies, too tired to do much else.

Since the first day that Steve was hospitalized, we'd barely kissed. We had little privacy in the hospital, and Steve felt so ill. The last time we'd made love was the morning Steve was admitted to St. Joe's, eight weeks before. So when Steve awoke with an erection one morning, I gently massaged him until he ejaculated a thin clearish fluid that burned his urethra. None of the chemotherapy information sheets mentioned sex. Nobody told us that chemotherapy destroyed sperm, or sometimes caused semen to disappear altogether. That dead substance, that watery ejaculate was off-putting. But I wanted to give Steve pleasure; his days were filled with anxiety, discomfort, loneliness. So I tried to arouse him another time. Again, the painful throbbing, the burning. After that, he pushed my hand away.

One night, as we lay next to each other in bed, Steve moved to caress me, but I couldn't bear it. How could I ask that of him, as tired and sick as he was, his last gasp of energy spent for my desire? How could I allow myself to feel pleasure when Steve felt pain almost constantly? "That's okay," I said, and moved his hand away. From the beginning our relationship had been intensely physical, lusty; in our lavender-painted bedroom alcove, our lovemaking was passionate and adventurous and fun. In sex Steve and I were joyful and synchronous, as we weren't always in other parts of our life. In the months coming, Steve and I would be more physically intimate than we'd ever been; I'd come to know his body almost as deeply as I knew my own, so close, so tender, but not through the act of love.

12. Zion

Thirteen days home, and then back to Zion. Steve tolerated his first round of chemotherapy well, so Dr. Sanchez decided to increase the dose of Adriamycin. Before they could begin, though, Steve underwent a routine exam. The doctors and nurses—different practitioners for the general exam—asked him the same questions, noted the idiosyncrasies of his body: the varicocele in his testicle (from Greek, *vein* plus *tumor*, though Steve's was benign and unrelated to his cancer). Lab technicians analyzed his urine and his blood, tallying lymphocytes and platelets—his body quantified, broken down into minute components, white blood cells counted like beads on an abacus. They examined every inch of him, inside and out, and Steve, the flesh and blood of him, what I could see and touch and lick and smell, became a collection of organs sheathed in skin, a mere body.

One entry on his medical records curiously referred to Steve as *she*: "Patient advised to be more active, which *she* is doing although *she* is still taking a lot of morphine and Dilaudid." An error in transcription, but disconcerting all the same, as if Steve had shifted genders. Latin distances physicians from actual humans, body parts translated into sterile medical terms. How else can doctors attend to dying individuals day after day without the buffer of jargon? But where is Steve in this passage? *Mediastinum normal; increased density of mid-thoracic vertebral bodies.* My interpretation: In the middle of Steve's back, that unreachable spot he asked me to scratch, the vertebrae—those hollow, bony lug nuts I pressed my thumb between when I massaged him, those lumpy rings through which bundles of nerves are housed like electrical wire—well, they'd thickened, which could mean the tumors had grown.

But I was not the doctor, the one with the knowledge, the years of schooling. I was the "friend," the "caregiver," the person whom nurses mistook for the wife: *friend at bedside*; *care giver knowledgeable and able to explain procedure*; *patient resting in bed with wife and watching t.v.*

The term *caregiver* implies a selfless, one-way relationship, but the role is more complex. Caregivers are takers, too. We give out of obligation, to avoid feeling selfish. We give to confirm our moral righteousness, because it is the right thing to do. More magnanimously, we give out of love, but our giving is a *loan* after all; in return we expect gratitude, or the promise of the gift returned in kind. The most virtuous motivation for giving is charity, expecting nothing in return, even enduring personal hardship or suffering: sacrifice. But sacrifice, too, seeks a return. Allegiance with god, grace. Giving, it seems, is the progeny of wanting.

My choice to assume the role of Steve's caregiver involved all these complicated reasons. (It was not a *choice* really, but an instinctive response, like jumping into a river to save a drowning person.) My role was as ambiguous as our relationship. Steve was dependent upon me, though he'd never officially asked for my help, and I'd never actually offered. Nor had we taken any vow: *In sickness and in health, till death do us part.* Still, many of the nurses assumed Steve and I were married. One night, a conscientious nurse named Michaelleana recorded my presence from the moment she came on duty, as if I were a patient too, someone to monitor.

1600: Wife @ bedside.

2000: Wife remains @ bedside.

2100: Wife remains @ bedside. Watching t.v.

2240: Wife remains @ bedside. No complaints offered.

No complaints offered. Was the nurse referring to me? To Steve? To both of us? At times, I felt as if Steve and I were one being, a compound patient, our love the tie that bound us: not blood, not law. But the body, its fragile periphery of skin, is the ultimate barrier between people.

Unlike Steve, I could take my body out of the hospital, and so near midnight, I did.

On this trip, I'd arranged to stay with a woman named Martha who'd advertised a room for the going rate, ten bucks a night, only when I arrived Martha was gone. Her son, Jeff, explained that she was a homecare aide and had been called away for the week.

"What type of work do you do?" I asked Jeff, who looked to be in his mid-to-late twenties, about Steve's age, with shoulder-length hair parted in the middle and scruffy sideburns zigging down his jaw line. He was playing chess on a small handheld computer.

"I'm a painter," he said. "Right now I'm collecting unemployment. I don't work for less than ten bucks an hour."

I disliked him immediately, collecting unemployment because he'd set a minimum price for getting out of bed every day, a wage far higher than mine.

"Who's in the hospital?" he asked, smoking a cigarette, stroking a puddle of gray cat in his lap.

"My boyfriend."

"Bummer," he said. "I'm trying to quit drinking. I haven't had a drink in over two weeks."

I noticed this: when you told people your boyfriend had cancer, they anted up their own pain and laid it on the table. At first, I thought it was generous, a kind of offering, but sometimes it angered me. Nobody's pain seemed equal to ours. I felt self-righteous and chosen, anointed and doomed at the same time.

Jeff showed me to my room, which I was certain was actually Martha's room, dresses hanging in the closet, knickknacks on the bureau.

The next morning, Jeff mixed a glass of lemonade, lit a cigarette, and resumed his chess game.

"I guess you like to play chess." I felt obliged to address this man in whose living room I was a stranger.

"Keeps me out of trouble," he replied. "I'm on probation for dealing drugs."

"Good luck," I said. *Wingnut.* For a moment anyway, it felt good to be mean.

Steve was less cooperative on this second visit to Zion. At admission, he'd spurned a rectal exam, a small revolt against his condition. He requested that the nurses lower the side rails on his bed at night, and grew bolder, asking them repeatedly to close his door. He had enough difficulty sleeping with Greg and Chuck snoring, vomiting, moaning, let alone the muffled talk from the nurses' desk. Steve requested that he not be woken in the middle of the night for blood pressure and temperature checks; a hospital is not a place to rest. Steve's insurrections may have been minor, but they added up to some sense of governance over his seditious body.

"I'm getting out of here," he said one afternoon.

The downside of the fractured dose chemotherapy was that for five days Steve was leashed to the intravenous fluids dangling on an I.V. pole, tethered like a dog in the backyard. The nurses were reluctant to issue release passes in the middle of chemotherapy, so that afternoon Steve reached up to the I-Med Infusion Pump, stopped the flow of the fluids, and unhooked the tubes from his chest.

"I don't think you'd better do that," I said. "We're going to get in trouble. This could be dangerous."

He ignored me. Why not? All risk was relative. Get in trouble? Scolded by the doctors? It was laughable. He might be dead soon. Exiting a side door, we escaped from the hospital unseen. It felt strange to be free with Steve. Usually, I was alone outside the hospital, the brick walls of the building the boundary between Steve's territory and mine.

The day was cold and gray, but the air was bracing, a tonic against the stagnant hospital air perfumed with the smells of bodies—sweat, urine, vomit—only slightly masked by antiseptic cleaner and the faintly biting sulfuric scent of medicine. Outside, we breathed deeply. We strolled on the sidewalk slowly like new lovers, held hands shyly as if we were dating. I liked Steve's hands, his long fingers, his palms still rough and callused though he had not worked in three months. His hands were large, but deft when he glued a part on a model car with Nate, coaxed an eyelash out of my eye, or clipped a barrette in Lisa's hair.

Since the onset of his illness, we rarely touched. His skin was tender, his liver—largest organ in the body—was bloated and hot, pressing against his abdomen. I was afraid of hurting him, so I offered only lambent kisses, short brush strokes. Sometimes even those were bothersome, like flies landing lightly, ticklish and annoying.

By the time we walked one block to the park, Steve was tired. We sat on a bench and watched a mother and a little girl standing on the shore of the small pond. The mother was absentmindedly handing bread to her daughter. The girl crammed fistfuls of dough into her mouth, every now and then flinging a crusts at the ducks. Steve laughed, and I kissed his knuckles as the girl filled her cheeks and her mother stared at something else across the pond.

Put your troubles in the hands of the Lord and he will help you. Steve tossed the card from his parents on the night stand, then reclined in his bed, tired from our excursion. I filled a plastic urine jug with water for the flowers. I checked selections on his menu card, marking off little boxes and circling breakfast options. I enjoyed this task; it felt productive and useful, polling Steve about what he wanted to eat the next day; it implied continuity, future.

I completed a dietary survey from the Department of Nutritional Services. Next to "Present Diet" I wrote: *organic fruits, veggies, whole grains, free range poultry, seafood.* Sanctimonious. Especially as next to "Previous Diet" I confessed: *mostly meat and junk food,* as if all Steve and I had dined on before were bacon cheeseburgers and Ho-Hos. I punished us for our bad behavior; we took a vow of holisticness. We were converts, zealots, forsaking our evil dietary ways and unhealthy lifestyle. Overnight, our entire diet changed. We no longer ate refined sugar, bleached flour or red meat, only organic food, which cost triple the supermarket brands. And no more smoking for Steve; he quit the day he went into the hospital, though the cancer cells ignored his lungs; it preferred his bones, to which it clung like barnacles.

All this concern about diet, but Steve couldn't eat anyway. He was slightly nauseated from radiation he'd had the day before. The radiologist, Dr. Mehta, had stopped by Steve's room to discuss the treatment beforehand. "This will help your back pain," the doctor had promised. Afterward, Dr. Mehta recorded the results: *The patient is feeling really good and there is no pain in the lumbar area. However, he has been having pain in the cervical spine area and I have a feeling we may have to consider treating the neck.* I liked that Dr. Mehta had used the word "feeling," a word that demonstrated sentience, someone who followed his gut instincts. He seemed a notch closer to shaman than technician.

Toward the end of Steve's stay, a psychologist, Ms. Forrest, taught him biofeedback, how to relax, to control those functions we typically can't, involuntary systems like heart rate and blood pressure. That seemed a daunting objective; I could barely control *voluntary* functions (mood, attitude, behavior). Tension exacerbated pain, so Steve had to relax, a strange notion given his circumstances. Ms. Forrest worked with Steve to maintain a positive attitude.

One afternoon, Steve and I attended a support group facilitated by Ms. Forrest. Along with a middle-aged man, I was the only family member among the dozen or so patients in a circle of chairs in a small conference room. Ms. Forrest handed us brochures titled: *I Can Cope.* She asked people to volunteer coping strategies, and so I outlined my "grand scheme" approach. "If something is bothering me, I ask myself, *What does this matter in the grand scheme of things?* That puts things in perspective." I was thinking of my complaints about my job, but nobody responded to my statement. I felt embarrassed after speaking, and realized only later how insensitive my comments were. Death *is* the grand scheme; nothing compared, nothing belittled death.

Friday night back at the apartment, Jeff was playing chess. The volume on the t.v. was loud, voices shouting from the screen. I mumbled goodnight, walked upstairs, crawled into bed and read for a while. I clicked off the light, but I couldn't sleep right away, never could. I stared at patches of light on the wall. The yellowish rectangles—light passing through panes of glass, shadow and candescence—were beautiful, unbidden. That's what we stood to lose in all this: beauty, or joy, the appreciation of beauty in its purest form.

Finally, I slept. Three or four hours later, that time of night when stillness is palpable—no wind, no cars or planes or people or birds, no dogs barking—I was awakened by a cat screeching, followed by Jeff laughing loudly. His guffaws sounded distorted, like in a tunnel, too loud for someone alone, I thought. My eyes opened wide, drawing in the dim light. I heard Jeff's maniacal laugh again, and the cat yelped painfully. I envisioned Jeff, the drug dealer, screwed up on hallucinogens, torturing the cat. I stared at the door knob burnished with street light, expecting it to slowly rotate at any moment, expecting Jeff to enter my room, rape me, carve me up with a knife, laughing that wild, enormous laugh the whole time. My body tensed with fear, all movement arrested, though my heart tried desperately to escape its crib in my chest.

Nights could be like that, scenes from frightening horror films. Disaster was no longer an abstract concept. Anything was possible and danger was everywhere. In the darkness, I couldn't differentiate the real from the imagined. In the darkness, I was always afraid.

13. There, There

At home, after our second trip to Zion, Steve was lethargic. His white blood cell count dropped by a third and had to be monitored weekly at the small hospital in Saline a mile from our apartment, a hospital I hadn't known existed. Illness had rearranged the world around us, moved landmarks to the foreground— hospitals, pharmacies, health food stores. In the morning, I cooked scrambled eggs, which Steve poked at. His mouth was sore and his sense of taste diminished, but he needed food to recover, nutrition. There was no pleasure in eating though. Involuntarily Steve lead an ascetic life, without epicurean pleasures, the lusts of the body: sex, food, tobacco.

After breakfast, I injected Steve's catheter with heparin, then removed the dressing and covered the tubing with plastic. In the bathroom, Steve placed a metal collapsible chair in front of the toilet, with a folded towel draped over the back, upon which he rested his head. He took a long time to pee, a side effect of the medications. I straddled the seat of the chair and kept him company. My hands and feet were always chilled, but Steve's body exuded heat like a thermal blanket, and so I'd place my cold hands on his hot back. I liked to feel the exchange of heat between us, the skin a conductor of intimacy, a small, sensual pleasure.

Before he showered, I gently massaged Steve's skin with a boar's bristle brush to chafe off dead skin cells, which opened his pores and allowed toxins to sweat out. Then he placed a plastic milk crate in the tub, an inflatable pillow set on top of it, and sat on this makeshift bench for a good half hour, his bony knees knocking together, scalding water soothing his body, which must have felt pummeled.

After, he dressed in his slinky silver jogging shorts (rayon or nylon or some lightweight fabric which offered no resistance), or the yellow, blue and red polka dot boxer shorts his cousin Jessica had given him as a joke. I settled him on the couch with his favorite afghan, the one his Grandma Nettie crocheted, and the remote control, his Dilaudid and morphine, throat lozenges, a pitcher of water and a glass, Kleenex, the phone, the egg carton of vitamins and jar of vitamin C powder, spoon— everything set on the coffee table within reach. I scrubbed carrots for his juice, watched him swallow pill after pill.

Around noon, I left for work, where for the next four hours I researched direct mail catalogues, wrote press releases, and talked with sales representatives. I never mentioned Steve at work, and if Phyllis or Kristin or Maggie asked how he was, I'd say, well, thank you, without adding any details because it was obvious from their anxious expressions that they didn't want details, and who could blame them? Besides, Steve *was* doing well. He'd surpassed the prognosis of Dr. Demmons and Dr. Linn at St. Joe's, which was two months. And he was not experiencing the typical harsh side effects of chemotherapy, the nausea and retching, the inflamed flesh at the infusion site. Steve never called me at work, and I rarely called him; I didn't want to wake him if he was sleeping, and the afternoons ticked by quickly.

On my way home, I stopped by Arbor Farms, a natural grocery store, to pick up vitamins or more carrots. I'd called around to see if I could buy organic carrots in bulk, but a fifty pound bag was too much. Where would I put them? Besides, I couldn't afford that many carrots at once. After taxes, my paycheck for twenty hours a week was about $140. I paid Sally rent, $250. She couldn't afford the entire rent alone, and I'd signed the lease. Since I didn't have health insurance, Cendra cost $25 a week. The rest of my paychecks I spent on food, gas, car insurance. I was down to dollars before pay day. Steve offered me money for food, but he didn't always remember, and I hated to ask. It seemed gauche, or at least awkward, to ask an ill man for money.

Steve was fortunate that his insurance covered most of the costs of his treatment, which were staggering. When his first bill arrived shortly upon our return from Zion, we gasped at the sum—twenty-five thousand dollars. Adriamycin, 5-FU, and Mitomycin cost between about $600 per dose—Steve used a bottle of each daily over the five day course. The hospital bed was $450 a day; we dreamed of the luxury hotel suite we could buy for that amount. X-rays and CAT scans and MRIs and radiation treatments added up to thousands. Aspirin or throat lozenges cost two and three dollars each. Ginger-ale, a buck. Enema kits and oral flushes were itemized, every disposable urine jug, every plastic bucket into which Steve spat.

On Fridays after work I saw Cendra. Quickly I forfeited the idea of recruiting Steve. Cendra brewed us both a cup of herbal tea, then plumped down in her easy chair, feet up on the ottoman, slurping a bowl of soggy cereal or yogurt. Her keeshond, Stella, pawed in behind her. Stella was an elegant creature, with her thick black stole and silvery streaks near her eyes. She didn't smell or drool or bark or lick herself, but quietly assumed her place on the rug.

If Cendra had a different pet, a growling, muddied, tongue-wagging, pouncing Labrador retriever, for example, I would have sought another counselor. I was at my emotional capacity and couldn't deal with paw prints on my dress or defend my crotch from a snout. By the time I landed in Cendra's office at the end of each week, I was ready to erupt. Her office was designed for this: a box of tissues within arm's reach, an overstuffed chair, thick-pile carpet to muffle sobs. I saw other patients while I waited, women who'd seen Cendra just before me or were waiting for another counselor. We entered looking anxious, exited sniffling. This was the place people came to unburden; we left lighter, dryer.

For most of my hour with Cendra I recapped everything that had happened with Steve and the hospital and my job. She was not the kind of counselor who only nodded and hmm-ed. She offered opinions and advice. She laughed and swore and responded soothingly. "There, there," she said softly when I cried, which was strangely comforting, though I found the phrase curious. *Where, where?*

Steve's parents called every couple of days but there wasn't much to talk about. Steve's dad said hello and handed the phone to his mother. Steve never had long conversations with her before, so that didn't change. Steve's sister, Linda, worked in Ann Arbor 20 minutes away, so after her shift, which ended at 3:00 p.m., she visited Steve once a week faithfully, usually before I was home from work or shopping. Karen, Steve's youngest sister, never called. A senior in high school, she was popular and busy. Likely she was unable to grasp the gravitas of the situation; I could barely grasp it myself.

I called Sally every now and then, but she eschewed long phone conversations (cars, phones, things mechanical were anathema to her, except for cameras). My mother phoned, and my other three sisters in Massachusetts checked in regularly, but they were a thousand miles away, and Steve and I remained in the back of their minds, our situation occasionally worrying its way into their consciousnesses for a moment before being displaced again by jobs and boyfriends and money problems and classes they were taking and mufflers that need fixing and errands to run, and besides, what could they do?

They sent cash and checks, which surprised me. I wasn't aware of the custom of sending money for the infirm; I never sent anyone money. I guess I never knew anyone who was seriously ill. My father sent $500, and my mother matched that, and my sisters and brothers sent money, even my youngest brother, Mikey, mailed $50, a week's pay from his after-school job at a gas station. Money mattered. Money helped. It was unclear, though, who the money was for. Steve was the one who was ill, but the checks were made out to me. I cashed them and spent the money (Cendra's advice). I needed it, though mostly for vitamins and health food and trips to Zion.

In the afternoons, Steve worked on stained glass projects. He was making two panels the size of rectangular cookie sheets, each with a large cross atop a hill, like Golgotha, one for his Aunt Ethel and one for his mother. He'd found a four-inch tall metal Jesus figurine in a thrift shop a while back, cast in some pot metal, weighty like a fishing sinker. The little Jesus was relaxed, his arms folded across his torso as if prepared for burial. Nevertheless, Steve soldered him back on the cross for good.

Steve napped periodically during the day, on the couch or the La-Z-Boy recliner. These and the bed were his stations, an invisible triangle whose points he shuffled to and from seeking comfort, or simply to move, to be in a different place, like a polar bear I saw in a too-small cage at the zoo once. Back and forth the creature padded, rangy and neurotic, scouring a path from one end of its cell to the other. But Steve was less mobile, enervated from the heavy dose of pain medicine. It was a trade-off; either he hurt or he was drowsy from the morphine. The science of pain management hadn't advanced much, it appears, since the Mesopotamians 5,000 years before Christ. They distilled opium as we do today. Morphine is a natural derivative of opium; Dilaudid is the synthetic. Both are narcotics, which produce stupor or euphoria, even coma, depending on the quantity.

Steve seemed clearheaded when he was awake, not euphoric by any means, but languid, sleeping twelve to fourteen hours a day. Morphine (Morpheus, the god of dreams and sleep) acts directly upon the central nervous system, relaxing muscles, slowing reflexes, depressing respiration. Listening to Steve breathe, I imagined an invisible weight, like an anvil, pressing down on his chest, preventing him from expanding his lungs, from inhaling deeply. His breaths were shallow dips into the ocean of air.

At night in bed Steve's body jerked and twitched while he slumbered, like a marionette on a string. His leg kicked out suddenly, or his body shuddered: myoclonus, a side effect of the morphine. It kept me awake, that and the need to pee four times a night, a sign of stress, though I was unaware of that. I assumed I had a never-ending bladder infection. I'd switch on each light in the apartment, skulking like a burglar from room to room until I reached the bathroom. I was afraid of the dark suddenly, perhaps because Steve slept so heavily that I felt alone, or because his body, with its twitching and jerking and sporadic grunts and whimpers made me feel like I was lying next to a stranger.

Or perhaps the idea of death had lodged itself in my subconscious. Every night I prayed for Steve to be healed. The last time I'd prayed (as opposed to meditating and chanting with Sufis and Sikhs at retreats in college) was in high school when I feared I was pregnant. I felt like a hypocrite praying. I didn't have any faith, but I rationalized that if there truly were a beneficent god, he'd forgive my intermittent worship.

In May, on a quiet Saturday when Steve was napping on the couch and I reclined in the La-Z-Boy watching television, I heard a tinny knock on our screen door and found Joey, Steve's childhood friend, standing on our veranda. "Hey Joe." I opened the door. "Steve, it's Joey."

Steve sat up on the couch, and Joey, looking scruffy in his leather jacket and shaggy hair, sat next to him. We were excited about a visitor, someone to take our attention away from each other, a live person, not a television show or movie.

"I saw your mother at Motor Vehicles," Joey said. "She told me about the cancer. Man, I couldn't believe it." Joey lit a cigarette. "How you feeling, buddy?"

"Pretty good," Steve said. "I was supposed to be dead by now."

Steve recounted his history, starting with the back pain, St. Joe's, Zion, the alternative treatments there, which he'd have soon, which insurance didn't cover. Steve was shirtless, and I helped him untape the gauze over the Infusaport implanted in his chest, above his right nipple but below his collar bone, which protruded from his chest like a mantle. Exposing his scar to Joey seemed a boyish act, a gesture of intimacy that had an air of innocence, indulging in curiosity about bodies. Scars promise stories of battles, of courage perhaps, or at least survival. Steve had told me that as a boy, he'd been jealous of kids with chicken pox marks, so he made his own. He'd removed the snub of pink eraser from the end of a pencil and pressed the hollowed aluminum tube into his flesh, cutting circles and half-moons on his cheeks and forehead, manufacturing scars in his perfect smooth skin.

"Mo's been researching experimental treatments," Steve told Joey. "She's got me on all these vitamins." He opened the egg crate with its clusters of pastel pills. Joey was quiet. I'd never heard him speak much anyway. I'd only seen him a few times since we first met, though enough to have altered my impression from suspicion to the kind of affection one has for the runt of the litter. Joey didn't seem to have much going for him. He worked at Hoyt's junkyard in the industrial zone of Steve's hometown, where flat-roofed, corrugated-tin warehouses occupied blocks.

A few months before Steve fell ill, he and I had searched for Joey at Hoyt's one night. Steve needed a radiator for his old jeep. The junkyard was surrounded by a chain link fence. Inside were piles of flattened cars, maybe five or ten cars stacked atop one another, and stack after stack as far as I could see, all the cars hopelessly smashed. Nobody was in the small wooden building at the entrance to Hoyt's, so Steve and I wandered toward the center of the junk yard. We stopped at a red convertible with its windshield fractured into tiny squares. The engine had been pushed into the driver's seat, the shape of a tree or pole formed in the hood as if the car were made of clay.

"That person couldn't have lived," I said to Steve.

Steve called Joey's name; it echoed, then a hush. The junkyard was still. There wasn't a living thing in sight. No birds. No bugs. Just dirt and metal and glass and rubber, an unpeopled city of wrecks and discards. We never found Joey that night.

Joey and Steve watched television for a while. In the mornings nothing aired except for talk shows, game shows, and odd sports like curling. But there was no need to talk or fill the silence. They'd known each other since they were kids, in Boy Scouts together, hanging around the neighborhood, launching UFOs on summer nights. To make UFOs, Steve had told me, they fastened a garbage bag to an empty soda bottle filled with kerosene they'd siphoned from Steve's dad's camp stove. Then they strung a wick through a cork and lit the contraption. The heat from the flame inflated the garbage bag, which would rise into the dusky sky and drift over the tall pines bordering Steve's house before extinguishing and falling to the ground.

Joey fished around the coffee table for some matches. He picked up the bell I'd set there, and jangled it. "What's this for?"

Steve and I smiled at each other. It was hokey, the little bell Steve was to ring if he needed something, though he didn't use it often. Sometimes he rang the bell wildly, then grinned when I arrived. *I missed you*, he'd say. Our apartment was so small that Steve only had to speak my name and I'd hear him. Even if I tried, I couldn't get far enough away for him to need the bell. But I placed a bell on the table because of my mother. She treated me and my siblings royally when we were ill, ordering my sisters to deliver dinner on a tray, permitting us to watch hours of television, drink soda freely, miss school and be exempt from chores—as a child, being sick was a vacation.

Joey picked up Steve's brown plastic pill bottle. "Dilaudid. Huh."

Neither Steve nor I questioned Joey's interest. We'd never head of Dilaudid before Steve's illness.

"These go for $40 a pop in the city," Joey said. "I might be able to get rid of a few of these, get you some cash. Can you spare some?"

"I guess," Steve said, twisting the cap and spilling tablets onto the coffee table. I didn't say anything because this didn't seem quite real; it didn't register. I wasn't capable of working out the ethics of giving Joey narcotics to sell, even if it was to help Steve. My focus was limited to each small unfurling moment, to the enclosed space of our living room, to Steve's diminished life, to his survival. I did not have the mental capacity for complicated moral dilemmas.

"Got a baggie?" Joey said.

I walked into the kitchen and returned with one. Joey scooped the pills into the baggie with the cover of a match book, counting them as he went along, leaving one pill on the table. He looped a knot in the bag and stuffed it in his breast pocket, then picked up the pill and walked into the kitchen. After a few minutes, I followed as I could hear him opening drawers. He pulled out a tablespoon and filled it with tap water. He dropped the Dilaudid into the water, and flicked a lighter underneath until the pill dissolved, then took a syringe from the box we kept on the kitchen table. (Steve had a prescription for a gross of syringes, which we used for injecting heparin into his Infusaport.) Joey dipped the tip of the needle into the liquid, drew back on the plunger, then thunked the syringe the way the nurses had taught me to do, to dissipate air bubbles.

I stood watching. I didn't really absorb what Joey was doing until he rolled up his shirt sleeve and tightened a bandanna around his arm, just below his bicep. Then he kneeled on the green and yellow flowered linoleum. I could see the top of his head, his bald spot, though his hair fell past his shoulders. He rubbed two fingers back and forth along the inside of his forearm, then pricked the needle into his vein and depressed the plunger, dangling a cigarette out of his mouth, crinkling his eyes against the curls of smoke. His movements were fluid and graceful, confident.

I'd never seen anyone shoot up and was aghast, but I kept quiet. Joey was so nonchalant about the whole matter, as if he'd helped himself to a glass of water. I walked back into the living room where Steve was laying on the couch, and in a while Joey followed.

"When you going back to Chicago?" he asked.

"Next week," Steve said.

"Take it easy, buddy," Joey said. "I'll see you in a couple weeks."

Joey and Steve shook hands in that soul-brother way, where the thumbs wrapped around each other, like a hug of hands. The screen door clattered. Steve raised his head to watch out the window and moments later Joey peeled away in a shiny red sports car. "Where'd he get that?" Steve said.

"Do you know what he just did?" I said. "He just shot up one of those Dilaudid. He used one of your syringes."

"Wow," Steve said. "He's worse off than I thought. Poor guy."

On Sunday, Steve's parents brought Lisa and Nate and Sarah to our apartment for the day. The kids were dressed up as they'd gone to church first. Lisa climbed up on Steve's lap as she was used to doing, but squirming around she accidentally pressed her hand on the catheter in Steve's chest, which yanked the tube. He winced, which frightened Lisa. She sniffled, her lip quivering. Steve soothed her, but after that she was shy about touching him. Nate and Sarah were reticent, too, witnessing their father's fragility, and so a new formality crept into their relationship; they kept a distance, having learned quickly, as I had, that Steve's body was off-limits.

By degrees, their father had left them. First separation and then divorce removed him from their daily lives, and now illness framed a buffer zone around Steve's body. Steve's behavior, too, was modified. He no longer tumbled with the kids on the living room carpet, raising Nate and Lisa in the air with his feet to fly like Superman, or transforming himself into a horse, letting them climb on his back to giddy-up. No more piggyback or shoulder rides, no more of Steve's silly walk. They didn't sit on his lap or snuggle into that warm place under his arm to read a book. But he touched them as they skipped by the couch, stroked them like you would a pony through a fence, and talked to them softly, exclaiming at the prettiness of the pictures they colored with crayons.

Nobody explained what was happening to Sarah, who at ten should have known more perhaps, or to Nate and Lisa who probably wouldn't have understood anyway. What Sarah and Nate and Lisa knew about Steve's situation was what they observed: their dad was sick, still.

Around dusk, Steve's parents packed up the car. The kids had to be home before dark as Sarah had school the next day. They kissed Steve gingerly on his cheek and said, "Hope you feel better, Dad." They buckled themselves into the back seat of Bill and Louise's car, and Steve and I waved to them from the porch as they headed west toward home, the sun foundering on the horizon.

Since Steve no longer exercised regularly, food bulked up his digestive tract. Morphine, a desiccant, caused severe constipation, which gave Steve stabbing abdominal cramps. Then we resorted to the enema kit we'd brought home from the hospital. Steve sat on the toilet, chin resting on his chest, back curved, me in rubber gloves with a jar of Vaseline, the plastic bucket and tubing, and it was like we were struggling with this *thing*, his body, this uncooperative and recalcitrant form. "Take a deep breath," I coached. "I'll be careful, I promise."

I spoke in a calm voice so as not to lend sobriety to the matter, so that we could consider this task ordinary like brushing his teeth. But we were in the bathroom for an hour, Steve was so anxious. Finally, after the third or fourth attempt, on an exhale, I was able to insert the plastic tubing, while warm water from the bucket I held above my head emptied into him. We were only marginally successful, but Steve had had enough. We'd try again tomorrow, or the day after.

In bed, I kissed Steve's cheek and he squeezed my hand a few times, like Morse code, then we rolled over to our sides. The locus of intimacy in our relationship had shifted, I realized, out of the bedroom, into the bathroom.

14. Cancer Man

O nce it was clear that Steve was not going to die any minute, we slowed down. That month, Steve and I drove to Zion, six hours by car but cheaper than flying. In Indiana time moved in reverse; we gained an hour. If we just continued driving west, I thought, earning hours like frequent flyer miles Steve would live longer, forever if we didn't stop. But we did, at the hospital, and Steve signed admission forms and checked into his room.

With a car, my range for accommodations was wider. I sat on Steve's bed and perused the yellow pages for hotels. The Harbor Hotel charged $75 a week, not much more than I'd paid in private homes. It was dark when I arrived at the Harbor Hotel (nowhere near any harbor). I rang the bell in the office, which was the living room of a small house that smelled of curry. In the background a boy played on the rug in the gray penumbra of the television. A woman wearing a sari, with a red dot on her forehead gave me a key. I wondered how she landed in this place, the Midwest. I imagined her arriving on the coast but not stopping, continuously moving to the safe middle of the country. The woman took my cash and pointed to a hand-printed sign: No Refunds. Then she directed me to my room, which was in their *other* hotel down the street.

A mile further west on the main drag, across from a block of nightclubs, I pulled into the parking lot of two-story brick apartment building, in its basement a dozen rooms. Leaves blew around the hallway. There was no front desk, only a broken pay phone, its receiver dangling near the floor as if a party were still holding on the other end, perhaps someone waiting to speak with the disheveled man who loitered nearby. The place was creepy, but not much worse than the sixth-floor walk-ups I rented while backpacking in Europe. The t.v. worked, sink, shower and toilet worked. The sheets looked clean(ish). I was spared from total disgust by the poor lighting.

Chuck was there, occupying the bed next to Steve. Occupy was the right word because Chuck never rose. Steve looked vigorously healthy compared to Chuck with his watery eyes, fluid breaths, flaccid skin. Greg was scheduled to arrive soon, too. Ramona and Sue and Estherine were back in the room across the hall. Steve flirted with them, bald and in their bathrobes. "I'm wearing my camouflage shirt for my upper G.I." he said, grinning in his mottled drab-green flannel.

Along with upper and lower gastrointestinals, which Steve hated (drinking chalky barium for the upper, the barium injected rectally for the lower), Dr. Sanchez ordered a series of baseline tests prior to the experimental procedure, whole body hyperthermia. A technician x-rayed Steve's chest to see if the cancer had migrated into his lungs (it hadn't), and computer tomography showed an updated picture of his bloated sick liver.

He was sent for another set of bone scans, which confirmed that cancer still occupied many posts throughout Steve's body: the calvarium, the fancy name for skullcap; the sacrum, that bony flange just above the coccyx; the lower portion of the hip bone called the ischium; and the acetabulum, the socket into which the thigh bone fits like a pestle in a mortar. Doctors of antiquity were poets; acetabulum in Latin means "little saucer for vinegar." There on Steve's little saucer, cancer grew.

The tests continued for two days. Steve fidgeted. On the second day, he signed a temporary release form, and we went out for dinner. We ate at Bob's Big Boy, bland food, bland people, except for the figure on the roof, the mascot: a chubby boy who was seven feet tall and probably weighed 500 pounds, wearing red and white checkered trousers with suspenders. What kind of logo was this? The other diners don't seem to notice how surreal the scene was, the waitresses with the "Big Boy" insignia patterned on their blouses as if they were members of a cult, their perky cheerfulness suspect. They can't be *that* happy.

"How's your fish?" I asked Steve. We'd both ordered from the heart-smart menu.

"It's alright," he said. "Doesn't taste like anything."

"The only fish that's safe to eat is orange roughy. Fish from cold waters off Australia." I'm full of facts from the health magazines I picked up at the natural grocer.

"What about Lake Superior?" Steve asked. "That's clean."

"Acid rain. Mercury. Pregnant women aren't supposed to eat *any* fish from the Great Lakes."

Steve and I didn't talk about anything important. We kept the conversation superficial: tidbits about people in the hospital, news about family and friends. We didn't mull over the past (our fights, breaking up), nor did we talk about the future. We didn't discuss the seriousness of Steve's situation. I never said, *Steve, I'm scared.* He never said, *I don't want to die, Mo. I'm too young.* We focused our thoughts outward. "Did you notice Greg never mentions his fiancé anymore? I think they broke up."

"She never calls him while he's here."

"Are your parents coming up this weekend?"

"I guess. It's crazy to drive all the way up here for one night and turn around."

Steve didn't say, *I miss the kids, I miss work, I miss making love.*

At night, Steve and I crammed into his hospital bed, and I read aloud while he rested. I recited poems or read clips about U.F.O.s and paranormal phenomena from *Omni* magazine, and stories from supermarket tabloids. For us these stories served a function; compared to the outlandish articles, Steve's situation seemed normal. GIANT FLYING CATS TERRIFY TOWN. WOMAN ABDUCTED BY ALIENS CAN NOW TALK TO ANIMALS. CANCER MAN'S LAST REQUEST: A JAGUAR CAR PARTS CATALOGUE. I envisioned a man in a leotard and cape with a big "C" on his chest, an action hero defying death. Cancer Man.

"That's a dumb request," Steve said. "Hell, I'd wish for the Jaguar." But he was speaking hypothetically.

The next day Cancer Man would undergo an experimental treatment, whole body hyperthermia. His body temperature would be raised to 108 degrees Fahrenheit. The theory was that abnormal, mutant cancer cells sloughed off at 107 degrees, while healthy cells—skin, organs, muscle, brain tissue—began to die at temperatures just above 108. It was a precarious balancing act to reach the right temperature, sustain it long enough to do specific damage, then lower it again.

The evening before the hyperthermia, doctors and nurses described the risks to Steve and me in affectless detail. "Yes, I understand," Steve said over and over, and a nurse recorded these exact words. Steve signed more forms: a Consent for Blood Transfusion, a Consent to Systemic Thermotherapy (Hyperthermia). Whomever wrote the permission slips had a biblical flair. On the Blood Transfusion form, this oath: *I covenant that I will never sue any of the parties specified above.*

The hyperthermia consent form—three pages of single-spaced text—listed more serious hazards than those of blood transfusion (hepatitis was mentioned, but in 1986, HIV was not). At the end of the form was a jarring litany of possible mishaps ranging from blisters, fatigue, diarrhea to nerve damage, foot drop, numbness in the fingers, blood clotting, lung or kidney failure. The conclusion: "Any one of these complications could result in death or disability, whole or partial, temporary or permanent." A curious syntax: the absence of a comma implied a possible return from death.

Dr. Kim said, "You are aware that a few patients have died from this procedure."

Steve nodded. "I understand."

The nurse jotted this down.

Steve initialed each page, and signed the last. With a scribble from a pen, he risked his life in an effort to save it. The final step was authorization from a spouse, guardian, or next of kin. A nurse phoned Steve's mother in Michigan. She was hundreds of miles away, but there I was right next to Steve, in bed with him, reading forms to him, flinching as a nurse injected valium into his arm, holding his hand through four excruciating enemas to cleanse his bowels, cooling his brow with a washcloth, but I could not sign, could not witness.

I was up at 6:45 a.m. on Thursday, our third day in Zion. The sluggish April sun was just rising when I drove to the hospital to see Steve as he prepared for the hyperthermia. I held his hand, kissed him goodbye, waved as he was wheeled into the operating room.

"I've done over nine hundred hyperthermias," Dr. Kim told me, his hand on my shoulder. He was a gentle, unassuming man, Filipino like Steve's other doctors. "Everything will be fine," he said. He must have seen fear in my face, mouth taut, a slight ruck in my brow. "Come back in an hour," Dr. Kim said, slipping through the swinging doors of the operating room.

The little chapel on the second floor of the four story hospital was empty, my own private church. It was dark, purplish, windowless, a dim garden of candles. I knelt at the altar and prayed, surprised that I could be that humble. I summoned the words to Our Father. Sunday Masses in childhood had lodged the prayer in my memory. I relished the quiet, tenebrous atmosphere of that grotto. Perhaps it was the smallness of the room, but somehow I didn't feel alone in there, or lonely anyway. After a while—who knows how long, time seemed unreckonable—I crossed myself. It was a reflex, these hand motions, and the words I spoke automatically. I listened to the susurrus of my whispered blessing: *In the name of the father, the son, and the holy spirit.* My Irish grandmother said holy ghost, but I was afraid of ghosts.

A nurse found me in the lounge at the end of the hallway on Steve's floor and delivered me to Dr. Kim in the operating room. Steve was lying on a table, relaxed with Valium, lulled to sleep with sodium pentothal, numbed by general anesthesia. He'd been stripped naked and wrapped head to toe in gauze like a mummy. Even his eyes were covered, which disturbed me. I pressed back tears.

"He can't feel anything," Dr. Kim said. That was not reassuring. A nurse tucked folded sheepskins under the points of Steve's body which pressed on the table: shoulder blades, elbows, heels. She placed a padded doughnut under his buttocks, layered on cotton blankets, more pads, more sheepskins.

"It will take four hours to raise his temperature," Dr. Kim said. "We'll keep it there two, maybe three hours. We'll see." He seemed unfazed by the responsibility before him.

"Okay?" he asked, as if he will not proceed without my signal.

I nodded and left.

The nurses continued the preparation. They wrapped Steve in a heated plastic blanket filled with 80% distilled water and 20% ethyl alcohol. The temperature of the water would vary from 120 to 140 degrees Fahrenheit, which would raise Steve's core temperature—the temperature at the center of his body—to 108 degrees, where it would hover for hours. Intravenous fluids would be pumped into his veins so he didn't dehydrate. All output would be measured. Nurses would carefully monitor Steve's temperature with a thermometer in his mouth, one in his rectum, one connected to the Foley catheter. The blood pressure cuff and electrocardiograph would track the beating of his heart.

On my way to the library a few blocks from the hospital, I spotted a jay-sized bird boldly garbed in a blood-red hood and black and white tuxedo, clinging to the side of a maple. A redheaded woodpecker. The bird stood out among the muted browns and greens in the park and felt like a gift, blatant beauty. I studied the woodpecker for a long time. It was so rare and striking, a blessing.

The library was decent for this small town. I spread out at a table and drafted a letter to Steve's insurance company, pleading with them to pay for the hyperthermia, $4,000 per treatment. I began with a rational approach: *From the information enclosed, it is obvious that hyperthermia is a valid treatment for cancer.* I continued in that vein, later blending in an emotional appeal: *Who knows when the major breakthrough in cancer treatment will arrive?* I wrote, as if it would be delivered any day by U.S. mail. *How tragic should a cure be discovered months after a death which could have been postponed with hyperthermia.* I was influenced by too many movies, the scientist in the lab shouting "Eureka!"—the cure arriving in a sudden, almost accidental breakthrough.

Steve and I had high hopes for the hyperthermia. It was our panacea, our godsend. The term "experimental" implies *anything* can happen, even the heretofore impossible. I remember an experiment in ninth grade chemistry: coagulation. We filled a pipette with egg white, applied heat. Presto. The substance changed from liquid to solid, clear to opaque, a complete transformation of matter. I envisioned the opposite in hyperthermia: Steve's tumors melting away, flushing out of his body through the Foley catheter.

I drafted another appeal, more emotional, directly addressing the insurance agents, rhetorically inviting them to step into Steve's shoes: *You are fighting the most relentless enemy imaginable. Everything is on hold: the house you wanted to buy, the cars you dreamed of owning, the classes you enrolled in.* That last part was for me, for the graduate school applications I'd filled out before Steve was diagnosed. Finally, I forced the insurance agents into Steve's situation, threatened like a malevolent god: *If it was you, your child, your loved one (and more than likely it will be as one in three Americans will get cancer in his or her lifetime)…*

I put the drafts aside. I'd read them aloud to Steve, see what he thought. I jotted down an idea for an exposé on the American Cancer Society (staid, conservative outfit—they wouldn't list hyperthermia as an approved treatment, though it had been practiced since the early 1970s): *How much money do they raise? How much goes to salaries? Who are these "decisive leaders" who determine what is "quackery" and what is not?* Years of reading *Mother Jones* had turned me into a Walter Mittyish investigative reporter. I had the ideas and the desire—I dreamt of being a crusader for justice, to speak for the disenfranchised—but I lacked follow-through.

Noon. Time moved swiftly, lost in my research, my writing. Steve had been in the operating room for four hours. His temperature had climbed to 108 degrees. I stopped in the cafeteria for lunch and saw Jane, who called me over to her table. She was a sixtyish woman with unruly white hair and huge blurry eyes behind thick glasses. I thought she was a volunteer when she walked into Steve's room the previous day and offered him a newspaper, then perambulated from room to room doling out carnations. But I learned at lunch that she was the mother of a patient.

"My daughter Bonnie is sick," Jane said. "She's thirty, my youngest of three. Got two kids of her own."

I'd never seen Bonnie leave her room, which was one door down from Steve's. Bonnie kept the divider pulled around her bed, the lights off, curtains drawn.

"She had a vertebrae removed from her spine so she can't walk," Jane said. "But she's doing better now that she's here."

Jane herself was robust. She had bouncy firm flesh, a full-moon belly, wide hips encased in stretchy nylon pants. She talked about her house in Iowa in painstaking detail: attached garage, kitchen with dishwasher, Cyclone fence around two full acres overlooking the Mississippi. She spoke in a flat nasally voice. "I have five dogs, two cats, a mallard which is now in my freezer waiting for the *Guinness Book of World Records* to verify it as the oldest albino duck—seventeen years, as old as my niece—and a pet blue jay that barks like a dog and shouts 'thief' every time a stranger comes in my house."

I was slightly embarrassed sitting with Jane in the cafeteria as she shouted about her life, but I was more annoyed that she chewed while she talked, projecting bullets of masticated bread. *Chew with your mouth closed*, I wanted to say, as my mother reminded me growing up. A slug of half-gnawed lettuce flew from Jane's mouth and landed on my cheek. It was all I could focus on. I gave Steve enemas, swabbed the raw, pink flesh around his catheter site, but none of that perturbed me the way having to eat with Jane seemed like an insurmountable task.

With my car, I could go anywhere. I drove to Lake Michigan and walked along the flat, pebbly beach, surprised at how dreary the Illinois shoreline was, not sandy and dramatic like the Michigan side with its massive dunes and turquoise water rolling shoreward in corteges of white-caps. A Chippewa myth about Michigan's Sleeping Bear Dunes tells of a mother bear and her two cubs escaping a raging forest fire in Wisconsin. They set out to swim across Lake Michigan, but along the way they encountered a storm. After paddling for days, the weary mother lumbered onto Michigan's shore and waited for her cubs. They never arrived.

From a canoe, the rising back of the dune resembled the silhouette of the mother bear in repose, still waiting for her cubs, the two Manitou Islands—South and North—which nosed out of the water a few miles offshore. When I first read that myth I felt inordinately sad. Something about the story struck me. Perhaps it was the beauty of the metaphor, or the artful storytelling of the Chippewa, their belief in numen, the ability to see breath and body in landscapes. Every time I thought of the story, I wanted to cry for the mother bear on whose back I'd climbed many times, whose body shifts in the harsh wind, yet she never stops looking. Zion's homely, shapeless coastline seems to have no story to tell, nothing to speak of its creation. Across the lake, I couldn't see the opposite shore or any islands, only a vast stretch of slate-gray water. I imagined the bears swimming. Unable to see the eastern shore, they must have forged ahead on faith alone.

I drove around, realizing quickly that there was little to see, the plain of water to the east, miles upon miles of cornfields stretching westward. Wisconsin was only twenty minutes north and I momentarily thought about driving there. Maybe Wisconsin was prettier, greener, and I could buy some of that cheese I'd seen advertised on billboards from Chicago to Zion. I imagined huge rounds of cheddar and Colby the size of cars. I'd bring home a wedge like a block of wood. But exploring the land of cheese by myself would be no fun.

Instead, I drove to a used book store in Waukegan, the small city bordering Zion, in a quest for Perry Mason mysteries, which Sally had turned me onto recently. When we were girls, Sally and I would rush home at 4:00 p.m. from wherever we were on summer days and sit in our cool basement watching the black and white reruns of *Perry*

Mason, starring the glowering Raymond Burr. I was enraptured by the show, and now I fell in love with the books, cheap little stories that completely absorbed me, simple words I could eat, pages I could bend and fold: *The Case of the Perjured Parrot*, *The Case of the Negligent Nymph*, *The Case of the Mischievous Doll*. I wanted to collect all 150 that Earle Stanley Gardner wrote, and kept track of which ones I'd read as if I were accomplishing something.

The mysteries reassured me. Perry Mason, inseparable in my mind's eye from the hulking Raymond Burr, always found the killer, always won his cases. I liked the surety of that. Reading those books blotted the screen in my mind; I temporarily deserted my life. In Waukegan, I hit the jackpot. Three titles I hadn't read before, only fifty cents each.

In the afternoon, I returned to the hospital. Steve had been transferred to the Critical Care Unit, which resembled a nursery (a wall of windows, crib-like beds with tall side rails). Steve was the sole patient. Two nurses continuously attended him. One nurse signaled me to enter. "He's a little restless but he's doing okay," she said. "You can see him for a minute."

I stood and looked down at Steve. He had an oxygen tube in his nose, an endotracheal tube down his throat to keep his airways open, a Foley catheter in his penis, and his subclavian catheter was hooked up to fluids. He was sweating rivulets; his breathing was labored; his eyes twitched under his lids. I witnessed. It was all I could do.

Steve woke an hour or so later, delirious, mumbling like a drunk, lashing out with his hands, wild and feverish, yanking at the tubes, trying to get out of bed. His brain was poached, addled with visions. He was likely having hypnagogic hallucinations: seeing things as if he were dreaming—falling, sinking, or the ceiling moving—but he wasn't asleep, just unconscious. Fevers over 104 degrees cause delirium, convulsions, sometimes coma. It took four hours to raise Steve's temperature to 108. It was going to take some time for his body to cool. The nurse bound Steve's wrists in restraints so he couldn't jerk his tubes out, and increased his valium.

Later, just after dark, I whispered, "Steve." His lids popped open, but he had dead eyes, fish eyes. They didn't focus or see, didn't follow light. He was only half there, half present.

I walked down the hall. The social worker saw me and paused. "You look like hell," she said.

"Thanks a lot," I replied. I understood that she dealt in truth, but I could have used a fib just then.

At two in the morning Steve woke, asked to use the bathroom, but he was still catheterized. The nurse explained this and he fell immediately back to sleep. A half-hour later, Steve was restless again, so more Valium. He woke at three a.m., wanted to use the bathroom. The nurse brought the bedpan but Steve wouldn't sit on it. He didn't know the condition of his own body, didn't know that if he tried to stand, he'd fall. Instead, he soiled himself. The nurse cleaned him up, and he slept, but soon he was awake again, still confused. The nurse gave him more Valium. Throughout the night, Steve had severe diarrhea. Nurses patiently diapered him. I was amazed that after four enemas he had anything left in his guts.

The next morning, Steve was alert but mildly confused. He had brain edema, so was retained in Critical Care. The nurses dosed him with Mannitol and Lasix to attenuate the pressure on his brain, diuretics which caused cells to forfeit excess fluid. Too much fluid in the body is as dangerous as too little. Pulmonary edema: one can drown on dry land. Late in the afternoon, Steve was transferred to his regular room,

321A. There, the problems were minor. Stomatitis: Steve's mouth was inflamed, possibly from the endotracheal tube. A nurse brought him a stomatitis cocktail: swish, swirl, spit.

"It feels like there's something in the back of my throat," Steve said to me, then to the nurse. "Something gets in the way when I swallow." Maybe it was the phantom weight of the nasal catheter, the way you feel a light band of pressure around your head after removing a hard hat. The nurse palpated Steve's throat, but couldn't feel any lumps—recorded "no mass on left or right"—as if Steve were imagining this closure of his throat, this dysphagia, but I suspected that what lodged in Steve's esophagus, what stuck and choked, was rage.

Steve suffered minor burns on his foot from the hyperthermia, and was slightly nauseated. I'd bought an electric hot-pot so I could heat soups I'd cooked at home, but the cream of broccoli I reheated smelled punky to Steve, made him queasy. He barely ate, threw up greenish fluid. And he had the runs still. His systems were amok, haywire. Doctors applied a pharmacopeia of remedies to right Steve's bodily malfunctions: Imodium and Kaopectate so he'd shit less; Mannitol and Lasix so he'd pee more. Benadryl and Seldane to dry out his water-logged cells; chloroseptic spray and Cepacol to moisten cotton mouth from damaged salivary glands; Zantac and Carafate to neutralize the acid in his stomach; Halcion to help him sleep. For Steve's fever, Dr. Sanchez ordered Tylenol, a 98-pound weakling compared to the powerhouse tag team of Dilaudid and morphine, narcotics Steve had been taking for three months. They were like old friends.

A nurse placed a vaporizer in Steve's room for moisture, which seemed primitive—heat and water—but perfect: steam, water wishing its way into air, a marriage of the elements, hydrogen and oxygen joining and separating and rejoining like partners in a waltz. I stood by Steve's bed or sat in the chair next to him all day, breathing in the vapors, my eyes closed to the hum of the motor.

At 8:30 p.m., Steve was ready to say goodnight. Back in my hotel room, I read for a couple of hours. The Harbor Hotel had been quiet all week. As far as I could tell, I was the only guest. Even so, I'd been sleeping with a light on, which I convinced myself was to prevent the cockroaches from crawling about, but which I knew was to ward off something else (ghosts, demons, spirits—my irrational fears).

Sometime later, I heard voices yelling and someone kicking the doors to the rooms, trying to crash one open. I distinguished two male voices, drunk, loud, and several other voices. They must have wandered in from the joints across the street. The voices moved progressively closer to my room. I clicked off my lamp so the intruders wouldn't see the sliver of light leaching out from under my door. I was afraid that if they found me, they'd kill me. It was my night-time logic. I ducked my head under the covers, practiced growling "Who's there?" in a deep, male voice. I made myself small like the tiny baby cockroaches that scattered for cover when I turned on the florescent light in the bathroom. I planned my escape out the casement window above the television, level with the ground. Luckily, the intruders managed to break into a room a couple of doors down. They partied there all night.

I slept as if drugged, woke to the sounds of Big Wheels on pavement. Lines pressed into my face from the wrinkled sheets formed a map. Outside, I blinked at the sunlight. Two young mothers sat on the brick steps smoking cigarettes. They stared at me as if I were an alien, out of my country, away from my land.

Chuck's bed was empty. "They took him out in the middle of the night," Steve told me when I arrived at the hospital. "He had a bad coughing fit. I don't think he's doing too well."

The day before, Chuck seemed to be improving, even sitting up and talking, breathing without oxygen for the first time in days. I walked downstairs to the CCU to find Sheila, to see how Chuck was doing, but neither she nor Chuck were there. A respiratory therapist figured out who I was looking for.

"He died this morning," he said.

"I thought he was doing better."

"We see that often," the therapist said, "a last surge of energy right before the person dies." A cruel trick, I thought, the body mocks the hope of the loved ones. Sheila was so optimistic when Chuck sat up. But maybe it's a gift, this eleventh-hour reprieve, a chance to offer a benediction: *God be with ye*, which, softened by centuries of spoken language, is just *good bye*.

Steve and I were surprisingly blasé about Chuck's death. We didn't grieve as much as wonder, pause. "Wow," Steve said. "Just like that." Steve was right. Chuck's death felt sudden in spite of his prolonged illness. I was sad for Chuck's wife though.

"Where's Sheila?" I asked the nurse on duty.

"She went home."

Gone without a trace, not one thread left behind. Chuck's bed had already been stripped and remade. Steve and I didn't associate Chuck's experience with ours, though. Somehow we felt like we were in an altogether different boat, sturdier, better built. To be perfectly honest, we didn't miss Chuck. The room was quieter without the chuff of the oxygen pump, the suck of the aspirator. And since we hadn't witnessed Chuck's death, or seen his dead body, it felt as if Chuck has just gone back to Decatur where he and Sheila were from.

Saturday afternoon, Steve's parents arrived from Michigan. When they saw my room at the Harbor Hotel, they were horrified. "Oh my goll!" Louise said, sidestepping blasphemy alphabetically, like saying dang for damn. "You're not staying here one more night," she announced, and I gathered my things quickly and they whisked me away to their nice, moderately-priced motel. We all slept in the same room, awkward, but more comforting and comfortable than the Harbor Hotel.

That night, Steve got a release pass and his parents treated us to dinner. Steve picked at his broiled chicken breast and succotash, separating out the lima beans. He didn't eat beans of any kind, and a host of other foods with a similar mushy consistency, like bananas or tapioca. I forked the lima beans off his plate, half-listening to his parents offering news on Steve's sister Linda and her husband, Kevin, the asparagus that was shooting up in Bill's garden, the traffic on the drive to Zion, the weather back home.

On Sunday, Steve asked Dr. Sanchez to start his chemotherapy. The sooner it was administered, the sooner Steve could leave. But he had to wait until his diarrhea cleared up, until he wasn't so weak. He could barely squeeze the nurse's hand during the strength test the day before. Steve's parents paid for me to stay at the hotel Sunday night, but I couldn't afford the room beyond that. There was an ad on the cafeteria bulletin board for a room in a house a few miles from the hospital. Helen, a fiftyish divorcée, had fixed up a spare room in her cellar with a comfortable double bed, a night stand, and lamp. There was even a private bathroom down there, though I had to walk through the scary section of the basement. Helen asked about Steve, and her unguarded reaction gave me pause. *Yes, it is sad,* I thought, lingering for a second on that sentiment, but not too long lest I got stuck there, the way my mother warned me as a child: *if you cross your eyes, they'll freeze that way.*

The last morning in Zion, I packed Steve's clothes and toiletries, and since we had the car, stuffed into his suitcase the egg-crate foam pad that was placed under his sheets to prevent bed sores. "This might be good for camping," I said. I packed the cheap, cut-glass, carnation vase from his night stand, as if it was a souvenir. We took a stack of small plastic, kidney-shaped basins, and pairs of disposable foam rubber slippers. Steve's insurance paid for them, so we were entitled. He owned them. The items weren't expensive or difficult to obtain or even necessary. They were worthless. But we were operating against the possibility of a still inconceivable loss, and so we vested material objects with an exaggerated value, as if the quantity and weight of our possessions would anchor Steve to this earth.

15. Motherlode

It's amazing how quickly a tectonic shift in a life can become routine. I pictured an arrow on a map: *You are here.* Suddenly a rumble, lightning, an act of God or nature or man altered the landscape. The change was something you lived with, like an in-law or cousin moving in. You made room (it demanded room). You molded your days around this change, incorporated the new thing into your life, even if the new thing was cancer. Mundanity crept back into each day: brushing your teeth, combing your hair, rubbing the sleep out of your eyes. Each ordinary hour blunted the jagged edges of the extraordinary thing. This was all that saved us from despair, from shipwreck. Momentum: the quiet forward motion of each day.

One night, Sally cooked dinner for us. "What are you making?" I asked Sally.

"I don't know," she said, opening the refrigerator. "Let's see what you have."

This made me nervous. What if the meal didn't taste good? Steve and Sally had been on tenuous grounds since they'd met, the awkward timing of her arrival in Michigan, Steve's assumption that I'd traded him for Sally, his resentment. But I'd forgotten that Sally was a sorcerer in the kitchen. When we were little Sally and I played restaurant. I'd drape a white napkin over my forearm in waiterly fashion. Sally, the chef, created hors d'oeuvres, which I'd serve to my younger sisters, Joanne and Barbie: white Wonder Bread spread with peanut butter, cut into inch squares and topped with a piece of Life cereal.

Sally had come a long way since then. She was the first female line cook at Chillingsworth, a four-star restaurant on Cape Cod. Later, she would be the chef at the Ingles House, a gorgeous stone mansion on the University of Michigan campus, where the university's president and board of regents entertained dignitaries. At the Ingles House, Sally would create dinners for Toni Morrison, Jaqueline Onassis, President Ford, Joseph Brodsky, Leon Redbone. That night, for Steve and me, Sally sautéed garlic, chopped onions and peppers, risking her fingertips with every staccato slice. She made cooking look dangerous: sharp knives, intense heat. The dinner was delicious, and Steve could actually taste the flavors. He complimented Sally, and thanked her, an olive branch between them.

Joey dropped by on a Saturday with his friend Phil. He'd never mentioned Phil before, but then again, Joey never mentioned any friends or girlfriends, though once when Steve and I stopped by his house, I noticed that his windows had dainty, gingham curtains and matching valences. It cheered me that perhaps Joey had someone in his life who cared enough to spruce up the run-down bungalow that he rented.

I unfolded a metal chair for Phil, who perched on it awkwardly, trying to find a comfortable or at least casual arrangement of his large, strong body. Joey reached into the pocket of his jeans and pulled out a thick roll of bills, which he set on the coffee table. Steve cleared a space on the table, unscrewed his vial of Dilaudid, poured out pills for Joey. Phil looked on, barely suppressing giddiness about Steve's motherlode of opioids, morphine and Dilaudid. Phil's presence seemed incongruous in our living room. He wore a sleeveless leather vest festooned with Harley Davidson insignia, had a pierced ear, a dagger tattoo on his bulked-up arm. I imagined that Phil accompanied Joey for the novelty of seeing a dying man, like a trip to the carnival to see the sideshow freaks. But the expression on Phil's face—feigned nonchalance—reminded me that Steve looked sick, his frame anorectically thin. You could count each rib and the knuckles of his vertebrae, trace the contours of his cheekbones and eye sockets.

Phil was telling a story. I don't recall the details. "So I told the guy to eat shit and die," Phil said, then glanced sheepishly at Steve, and mumbled, "Oh, uh, sorry," though Steve hadn't reacted. Phil's self-conscious apology for uttering a conjugation of the verb *to die* only created more awkwardness, as if the word itself had the power to kill, as if he'd reminded Steve of what was impossible for him to forget.

When Steve was up and about, we drove to his parents' house. Nate turned five, so we had a party for him. Louise baked a chocolate sheet cake with blue-icing letters. Someone picked up Grandma Nettie from the nursing home. Steve's cousin Jessica and her husband, Fran, along with Steve's Aunt Ethel, his sister Linda and her husband, Kevin, circled around the table as Nate sucked in a mouthful of air. Lisa mimicked Nate, stretching her mouth wide, and they both blew out the candles, spraying saliva and wax over the frosting.

"I think I'll pass on the cake," Kevin said, and everyone laughed.

Sarah leaned across the table, waiting for a slice. Her hair had grown long, reaching half-way down her spine, a pretty strawberry blonde. She pulled strands from the front and clipped them back with a barrette, so grown-up looking.

Steve gave Nate a robot toy, which lit up and stepped stiffly across the dining room table, along with a baseball glove. In the backyard, Steve and Nate stood six feet apart and tossed a ball back and forth. "That's good," Steve said, whether Nate caught the ball or not. Later, the kids played on the swing set in the backyard. The men watched a ball game on t.v., and the women talked around the dining room table. "Kevin's being laid off," Linda said. "We don't think it'll last long this time."

"Bill's doing piece-work," Louise said. Bill earned eight dollars for every door frame he built, so he had to work fast and hard to make money. It saddened me that Steve's father scrambled to earn as little as I did. Grandma Nettie sat quietly in the rocking chair in front of the huge picture window which overlooked the back yard. The window was custom-made, nearly floor-to-ceiling and wall-length, clear enough that you might walk straight through it, if not for Jesus hanging on Steve's stained glass cross, suspended by filament from the window frame, casting beams of red and pale purple light into the dining room, reminding you of barriers.

Outside the kids swung and ran and slithered down a tiny slide, Sarah's orange hair flying and Lisa's arms flailing, Nate's legs pumping as he lifted higher and higher on the swing. The kids were shouting or singing, but soundlessly on this side of the window, which reminded me of watching tropical fish in an aquarium: peaceful.

Later, Jessica brought out an old blonde wig she'd found somewhere and gave it to Steve as a joke. Steve plopped the fake hair on me, and I posed for a glamour shot, my head tilted rakishly. In the photo I am smiling, maybe on the verge of laughing. Anyone viewing this snapshot now—as a historical document, a piece of evidence—could infer that I was happy and having fun. That's how photos tell the truth and lie: in spite of my life beyond the borders of the photo, for that fleeting moment, I *was* happy.

"Try on the wig, Steve," Jessica said, and he relented. I captured him on film before he could protest. With that yellow-haired wig, his moustache grown back, smiling broadly enough to dimple his cheeks, Steve almost looked like his old self.

16. Case of the Nosy Neighbors

Steve suspected that our landlord, Melissa, who lived below us, or else her two boys, one a teenager, one pre-teen like Sarah, were entering our apartment while we were gone, so before we left for Zion this time he set traps: little scraps of paper on doorknobs, which would flutter to the floor like moths if disturbed; trip wires of sewing thread across thresholds; talcum sprinkled lightly on the floor. It was like a game, this espionage, the type of subterfuge that Perry Mason might engage in: *The Case of the Nosy Neighbors*.

In the admissions checkup, the doctor told Steve that his white cell count had doubled since the last chemotherapy, a healthy return, but his hemoglobin was low. Hemoglobin delivers oxygen to body tissue, so Steve was slightly oxygen deprived. Doctors shored up Steve's blood with two units of packed red corpuscles, and I was grateful that somewhere someone had donated blood, an act of love for sure, to give one's blood to help a stranger.

The doctor gently rapped on Steve's torso with a tiny rubber-head hammer to measure the girth of his liver, which was slightly smaller than before: a positive sign. A nurse checked his blood pressure, and the doctor eavesdropped on Steve's chest, listening for the lubb dup of his heart. To be treated with hyperthermia again, Steve could not have heart irregularities: no *thrills*, which can sound like soft blowing or conversely, loud booming; no *gallops*, in which the heart beats thrice per cycle, one extra pump, resembling the gait of a horse; and no *rubs*, friction caused by an inflamed membranous sac chafing against the heart.

During hyperthermia, Steve would be wired to an electrocardiogram, which monitored the heart's electrical activity. Electricity keeps the body going, keeps the heart pumping, energy that cannot be created or destroyed. Strange. What force ignites the current inside us, I wondered, what keeps our hearts ticking every minute of the day, week in and week out, year after year like a metronome, a perpetual motion machine, two and half billion beats in an average life span? We take the heart for granted. We don't even think about its ceaseless activity, its singular indefatigable mission on our behalf until we're in love and our heart is fluttering, or we're frightened and it's pounding.

I drove to Helen's house. Jane from Iowa, mother of Bonnie, had beaten me to the better room—the room with a door that locked and real walls—but Helen's son had rigged a makeshift camp in the open part of the cellar, a couple of shower curtains on a track, which enclosed a space just larger than a double bed. Helen placed a night stand in my little hiding place, with a lamp set on a doily, a homey touch.

"Oh, you're here too," Jane said. She confided that she was concerned about Bonnie, feared that Bonnie had lost her will to survive. "There's no way I'm going to let her die," Jane said. "My son-in-law's got his job and two kids. I don't know how much longer he can do this. And he needs his wife. A man's gotta have sex." Jane talked on, standing near my bed in her long flannel nightgown. Exhausted, I half-listened, waiting for an opportunity to break in and excuse myself. Still, I was relieved that Jane was with me in the basement. I felt safer knowing she was lying in her bed ten feet away from mine, her snores resonating through the thin sheetrock.

I climbed into the bed in my strange encircled space, and clicked off the light. The chiaroscuro of the basement transformed the shower curtains into swaying figures, until I fixed my eyes steadily on them and willed them to be curtains again.

In the morning, the nurses reviewed the risks of hyperthermia with Steve. "This is my second hyperthermia," he said, a gentle reminder that they needn't fuss. "I know what to expect this time." But I wondered: if he knew what to expect, how could he endure it again?

Steve passed a rough night in the Critical Care Unit after this second hyperthermia treatment. He had pulmonary edema, fluid in his lungs, and hypoxia, oxygen deficiency, which purpled his fingernails and lips. The nurses placed an oxygen mask over his face, but in his delirium, he kept trying to rip it off. Dr. Kim stood at Steve's bedside frequently, and Dr. Sanchez, too. They ordered a chest x-ray, which showed clouds of fluid in Steve's lungs, the lower lobes filled with thick mucus. Fearing pneumonia, they retained him in Critical Care.

Pneumonia was a frightening specter in my childhood. My mother would say, "Get inside or you'll catch pneumonia. You'll catch your death of a cold." When I was three, I'd been hospitalized with pneumonia, as had my sister Joanne. And I knew that many cancer patients, their immune systems dangerously depleted by chemotherapy, died not of cancer, but pneumonia. Pneumonia, that bad cold, is the eighth leading cause of death in the United States.

Three days after hyperthermia, Steve was still coughing up yellowish sputum, and x-rays showed a spot of pneumonia on the lower right lobe of his lungs. Dr. Sanchez prescribed antibiotics and the respiratory therapist gave Steve a nebulizer treatment. The therapist brought Steve a spirometer to strengthen his lungs, a small plastic device that looked like a toy. Steve was to blow into the mouthpiece and elevate tiny ping-pong balls. The more balls Steve raised, the higher they floated, the greater his lung capacity.

Steve blew; he raised two balls. He had to raise four before they could start chemotherapy. He set the spirometer on the night stand after the first day, and left it there.

"You're supposed to do this five times a day," I said.

"I don't feel like it," he replied, his first sign of malaise.

The respiratory therapist and the doctors and nurses urged Steve to blow. Five days passed and Steve still had lung edema. I tried the spirometer myself, as if my effort could somehow help Steve. I found it surprisingly difficult to raise the balls, and I understood why Steve was discouraged. The spirometer made you feel like a failure at something as basic as breathing.

Louise visited on the weekend. She and Steve played cards endlessly, or they paced the hallways. I sat on an empty bed in Steve's room, logging hours for work, or reading Perry Mason mysteries. As always, the television was on in the background. I was glad for Louise's company, glad that Steve had someone else to help keep his mind off his body, though that was a difficult task. A week after the hyperthermia, Steve began to complain of pain in his lower back and hip. Oddly, the bone pain was a positive sign. Steve had the strength to complain, which indicated a return to normal, or what had passed for normal for four months.

At home, when we stepped into our apartment, we saw the results of Steve's espionage: paper scraps on the carpet, threads broken, the powder mucked by footprints. "I knew it," Steve said. He was worried about his lockbox of cash, the down payment he'd saved for a house, and money he'd been socking away for the experimental hypothermia treatments, which costs $4000 each. His union had raised $2,000 from a raffle of tools they'd organized on his behalf; he had the drug profits from Joey; and $4,000 his parents' church had raised through two soup suppers. I imagined all those good church-going strangers paying a few dollars to eat soup, helping to save Bill and Louise's son. I visualized the cauldrons of soup needed to raise $4,000, then I figured they must have served other foods, it was just *called* a soup supper. All that cash was locked away in Steve's shoebox-sized safe underneath a pile of steel-toed work boots and sneakers.

In a week, when Steve felt better, he'd change the locks.

I returned to work. Kristin had quit; she'd taken a job in a bookstore. Less pressure. Phyllis hired a new administrative assistant, Monica, a fiftyish woman with graying hair, heavy-set and watchful. She kept a stockpile of food in her desk drawer, which she nibbled on throughout the day, perhaps to give her energy to fight what appeared to be chronic exhaustion, every task accompanied by weary, audible exhales. At first, Monica was friendly as I showed her how to process orders. But after a day or two she resented my overseeing her work, so I left her alone.

Phyllis's business was growing, and so she leased a building for her company. One day we packed boxes and moved out of her basement into small office building, which was sunny and bright, with a patch of grass outside. Phyllis hired a shipping manager, Rebecca, who at twenty-six was a year older than me. She was tall and thin, with a master's degree in music.

"Do you play violin professionally?" I asked her.

"Rarely," she said. "I have tendinitis in my elbow."

"Oh, how sad." I assumed that someone who'd invested in so much training would be crushed at the loss.

"Not really," said. "I don't have much interest in performing."

I was relieved. I couldn't bear any more tragic stories.

My desk was adjacent to a window and a lovely breeze snuck in and caressed my arms at unexpected moments during the afternoon. The landlord's son, Frank, mowed the lawn weekly, waving when he saw me watching out my window, sometimes idling over to chat. His face, sieved by the screen, appeared rough, elusive. These visits, though pleasurable, made me anxious. What if Phyllis saw me lazily hobnobbing this way? She wouldn't say anything probably, but I'd detect disapproval in the way she'd avoid eye contact, the deliberateness with which she'd shut the French doors to her office.

Frank's wife, Greta, reconciled Phyllis's books twice weekly. From Germany, Greta was fair, with a delicate nose and deep-set blue eyes. Her precise pronunciation and sing-song inflection turned English into a new language, delicate and euphonious. Listening to her speak was a small pleasure. Greta was kind-natured, as was Rebecca, and it seemed as if Phyllis had hired me friends. Though I didn't socialize with Greta and Rebecca on weekends because of Steve's situation, we ate lunch together on the grass in the shade of an apple tree. Coincidentally—or maybe not given the incidence of cancer—both Rebecca and Greta had lost their mothers to the disease, Greta only months before, Rebecca when she was sixteen. They weren't apprehensive about discussing Steve. One day I told them that I was afraid that if Steve died, I would see his ghost and be terrified.

"My mother's spirit came to my room one night just after she died," Rebecca said. "She sat on the end of my bed, but I wasn't afraid. I was happy to see her." Greta believed that if you were not open to receiving spirits, they wouldn't visit. I liked that concept, that if the time came, I'd have a choice.

Frequently, Steve urged me to resign from my job, and I wanted to quit so that he wouldn't be alone all afternoon, but I was saving that option for when he *really* might need me. He wrote me a letter. *I need and want to be with you now, not when or if I get worse.* His favorite part of the day, he wrote, was when I came home from work, the bustle of unloading groceries, cooking dinner, chatting about my job. Aside from occasionally walking a half-block to the stained glass supply store to pick up copper tape and chat with Betsy, the owner, or a weekly visit from his sister, Linda, Steve spent most of each day alone.

My counselor, Cendra, strongly advised me *not* to quit my job, to maintain contact with the outside world rather than immerse myself completely in Steve's life. She suggested I see Sally once a week.

"I'm meeting Sally for a beer after work," I told Steve one day.

"Is it really so important to go out for a beer?" he said.

"She doesn't know that many people," I replied, converting my need into Sally's. Sharing a beer with my sister seemed frivolous given Steve's situation, but part of me was relieved that Cendra had given me this permission to get away for a little while. Against my sense of obligation and guilt (guilty for leaving Steve, guilty for neglecting Sally, I felt guilty all the time), against my love for Steve and concern for his well-being, I abided a faint throb of desire, an impulse toward self-preservation, toward my own life.

One weekend, Sally invited Steve and me to a barbecue, along with Evie, a baker with whom she worked, and her husband Chet, a social worker. Steve was reluctant.

"It's beautiful out there," I said. "It will be good to get out." After some cajoling, he finally agreed.

I gave Steve a quick tour of Sally's apartment, which was technically mine too as I was still paying half the rent. "It's a little small," he said.

"But isn't it nice?" I pointed to the brick hearth and wood stove, the view from the kitchen window, which overlooked a pond. Sally had shot Polaroids every week from that vantage point, looking down upon a small creek that fed into the pond. She'd hung the photos in succession on the wall. In the first shot, a smooth white blanket of snow cloaked the topography. In the succeeding photos, the snow shrank to a slushy mantle, the creek identifiable as a depression in the grainy surface, pierced by tufts of pale dead grass. Then the snow melted completely and the creek was darkly visible, but the world was still black—tree trunks and leafless branches and flattened cattails. Finally the snapshots looked exactly like the view out the window on that day—the creek gurgling into the pond, marsh grasses springing from the embankment, new curls of maple leaves unfolding like tiny hands.

It was fascinating to see time move so quickly in the photos, yet arrested completely: to study the evidence of change and renewal. It restored my faith, which wavered every winter, a perennial amnesia. Just when I was convinced that winter would never end, that the gray days would persevere monotonously, the thermometer fixed at cold, just then warmth and light lilted into the days and birds arrived as if by invitation and water freed itself and peepers trilled and wind sighed across hay fields.

Sally and I prepared food while Steve talked with Barb and Chet on the deck.

"He looks awful," Sally said, crying as she arranged crackers on a tray, wiping her eyes on her festive, thrift-store apron, patterned with green olives floating whimsically in martini glasses. I'd barely noticed the small incremental changes in Steve's physique; I hadn't registered the cumulative effects of his disease. But Sally, who had not seen Steve in weeks, was as surprised at his appearance as I was at the view outside her kitchen window. I hadn't registered until then that spring had arrived.

At home, Steve sat on the toilet, resting his head on the fold-up chair. I massaged his back, daring to touch him because he was feeling better after the last treatment, had more energy, perhaps because of the hyperthermia treatments, perhaps because three weeks had passed since this last chemotherapy instead of the usual two, so his body had rebounded. I walked my fingers along his spine, pressed the fleshy pad of my thumb in the hollows between his vertebrae. "I think I feel a tumor," I said.

"What does it feel like?" Steve asked.

"Like the bone, only shaped differently, off to the side. It's where it shouldn't be." I retraced my fingers over the nodule in case I was mistaken, in case the lump had disappeared somehow, but there it was, others too.

Once when I was alone in an elevator, out of curiosity I closed my eyes and touched the braille numbers on the panel with my fingertips. I couldn't make sense of those bumps, but my fingertips floating gently on Steve's skin distinguished the dorsal ridges of his vertebrae from the tumors lodged along his spine. "What do they feel like to you?" I asked.

"I can't explain," Steve said. "But sometimes they hurt so bad, it's like taking a piece of glass and cutting into the tip of your finger."

"The pain is sharp?" I was surprised.

"It's sharp and dull," he said. "It pounds, but it's steady. It's there all the time."

I circled my palm lightly over his back, drawing wider and wider moons, craving to press hard, to really touch him, to blanche his flesh with palm prints and watch them rouge.

Before Steve was ill, on nights when he and I were alone, we gave each other full-body massages. We spread towels on the living room floor and heated baby oil in a teacup in our microwave. We spent hours caressing each other, attending to all parts of our bodies—toes, knees, buttocks, biceps—sliding our warm hands in warm oil across the frictionless plain of skin and muscle, relaxing and soothing and melding into one form as we languored into patient, attendant, sensuous lovemaking.

When Steve was healthy, we made love nearly every day: mostly in the mornings, hurriedly on weekdays before work, quietly on weekends if the kids were sleeping in the living room. Instead of starting each day with a prayer or meditation, Steve and I worshiped the temples of our bodies, abided the creed of desire. It didn't matter if we'd fought the night before; we couldn't resist each other's flesh, warm and sour and salty. Steve was a gentle lover, curious, tender, fully present. In bed, we were generous to each other in a way we were not always otherwise. Making love, we were our best selves. That's what I missed most about my relationship with Steve, the union of our bodies.

17. Dunleavy Lane

In June, we celebrated our birthdays, which were two weeks apart. Steve turned thirty; I turned twenty-six. I bought Steve a goose-down pillow so soft and luxurious it smelled of sleep. The pillow cost a third of my weekly paycheck, but the difference between that and the cheaper grade was obvious. The goose-down pillow was stuffed with the finest white fluff from the breast of the bird, which warmed fragile eggs in the nest, where the goslings huddled once hatched. That was the pillow I was compelled to buy for Steve to place between his knees at night, to prevent the pressure of bone on bone.

I was surprised that Steve had a gift for me. He so rarely left the apartment alone, but he must have ventured out while I was at work one afternoon. I pictured him walking around the mall in his droopy jeans and brown leather cap, trying to find the right gift, resting alongside the senior citizens on benches. He bought me a jewelry box, which perplexed me. I didn't have any valuable jewelry to speak of, only vintage costume jewelry, like the ring with a lavender, hexagon-shaped cut-glass center, surrounded with seed pearls and rhinestones, heavy as a marble but worthless.

The jewelry box was an elaborately crafted miniature armoire that stood a foot-and-a-half tall. On one side were two tiny etched-glass panels with gold-plated knobs, like little French doors that opened to a closet with hooks for necklaces. I filled the elegant box with my unworthy baubles and set it on my dresser. I didn't have much occasion to wear jewelry anymore, and so the box would be untouched, like a museum display case, a reliquary for objects from a bygone time.

In late June 1986, Steve and I returned to Zion for his six month evaluation. For three days Steve endured tests: bone scans, brain scans, scans of his abdomen and pelvis, the gastrointestinal series. He began another round of chemotherapy as we waited for the results. On day four, Dr. Sanchez walked into Steve's room and stood with his chart at the foot of Steve's bed. "I have good news," he said.

Steve propped himself up on a pillow, and I sat on his bed.

"The cancer is stable." Dr. Sanchez smiled, awaiting our response. Steve was silent.

"What does that mean?" I asked.

"It means that there are no new tumors."

"What about the other tumors?" Steve asked.

"They're the same. No growth." Dr. Sanchez was pleased. He must have enjoyed those rare days when he could deliver promising results to his patients, nearly all who'd been diagnosed terminally ill at other facilities and had come to Zion for the experimental treatments, the holistic approach.

"I just wanted to give you the good news," Dr. Sanchez said, leaving us with a moment of privacy. As the door closed, Steve said, "That's not good news."

"Yes it is," I said, then paused. "What were you expecting?"

"I was expecting clear scans." Perhaps someone on Steve's medical team should have been more explicit about what was possible given his advanced disease, so that Steve's expectations weren't wildly out of the realm of reality. I had hoped for some reduction in the tumors, but I knew the outcome could have been worse.

"The cancer has stopped growing," I said to Steve. "They've stopped one of the most aggressive cancers known."

"But look what I had to go through!" he said. Homeostasis was not good enough for Steve, who expected more of a cure for the price he'd paid in suffering.

Two years before, on that day Steve and Joey and I had browsed through their high school yearbook, I'd seen a photo of Steve in his track uniform. He'd competed in his junior year, but quit after one season. When I'd asked him why, he'd explained: "I worked so hard. I ran miles after school for weeks and weeks. I ran as hard as I could. The coach about killed us." I'd visualized Steve's long legs striding nimbly along wooded trails, propelled by pure muscle, light and swift like Mercury with winged heels. "When we finally had a meet, I came in second place," he'd told me. "That's good," I'd said. "So why did you quit?" I remember Steve's incredulous look that day. "I'm not going to work that hard for *second place*."

Back then, I saw in Steve a quest for perfection, an unwillingness to accept less: all or nothing. I'd admired that he had high standards. But now the race was for life itself: *all or nothing*. I wished he'd settle for runner-up, or the modest gain he'd made so far.

Just after Steve's six month check-up, my lease with Sally for 11505 Dunleavy Lane ended. Sally was moving into a tiny house closer to town, a one-bedroom, asbestos-shingled bungalow a short walk from the Huron River. Sally's house was no more than a shack, but it presided over a stately lawn bordered by a hedge of lilacs. Steve assumed that I would officially move back into his apartment in Saline, where I slept every night, where I had my clothes in the dresser, my comb and brush on the bureau, next to the elegant jewelry box. I discussed my options with Cendra.

"I'm worried that if I move back in with Steve and he's cured, I'll just have to move out again because we never resolved our problems."

"Uh huh," Cendra said slowly. I could tell from her tone that she doubted Steve would be healed. Even so, she urged me to maintain my independence. Since the rent at this new house was half what I'd paid at Dunleavy Lane, I decided to sign the lease and share the house with Sally, in spirit if not in body. I wrote Steve a carefully articulated letter reminding him that I'd moved out for a reason, our relationship problems, which we'd never actually resolved. I sounded prudent, not urgent and heady like my letters to him early in our relationship. *We can't live on love alone*, I wrote, as if love were a food group, a carbohydrate, or a sugar: sweet, but unhealthy as a steady diet.

"I don't see why you are paying rent to Sally when you are living here," Steve said. "It's stupid." For days he stewed. And then almost overnight, it seemed, he turned angry. He felt betrayed by my decision, betrayed by his own body after six months of treatment, and his sense of betrayal was compounded by his daily discomforts—sore mouth, inability to taste, numb fingers and toes, burning urination, pain along his spine—and the sheer frustration of being perpetually sick, the continuing alienation from life outside of his apartment, from a place as small as Saline or as big as the world beyond, this compote of pain and frustration percolated inside Steve and manifested in a boiling anger palpable to doctors and nurses and everyone around him, but which he vented mostly toward me.

One night I reminded Steve that I'd be home later than usual since I was meeting Sally after work. "Don't bother coming back," he said. When I returned later that evening, he said, "I told you not to come back. I don't want you here."

I refused to believe him. "Who's going to cook you dinner?" I said, which only emphasized his dependence.

"I don't need you," he said.

"Yes you do," I insisted.

I needed him to need me. How could I be kicked off the project of helping save Steve? How could I live with myself if I left Steve suffering alone? The more I persisted in declaring Steve's need (thus his weakness), the angrier he grew. At times, he simply refused to speak to me. He drank the carrot juice I brought him, swallowed the vitamins I arranged, but he wouldn't let me touch him, wouldn't acknowledge my presence. When I said, "I love you," each night before sleeping, he didn't reply.

Anatole Broyard, who suffered from cancer at aged seventy, wrote that "every seriously ill person needs to develop a style for his illness." Broyard's sanguine disposition seems the luxury of an old man who's lived a good long life, but there's some truth to it. Outwardly, Steve was mellow, which disguised an undertow of passion and intensity. This duality had drawn me to him when we first met in New York, his soft, almost boyish voice and visage, his tender touch opposing physical strength, tensile stubbornness, drive and determination.

In illness, Steve was the same as he was in love, in life. At first he was calm, focused, optimistic. But then his anger, which had been quietly simmering, exploded. One night I carried a plate of dinner to him in the living room. He ate a few forkfuls, then spit out the food. "This tastes like shit!" he said, sweeping his arm across the coffee table. The plate sailed into the air, bits of fish and potato spraying across the floor.

"I'm not picking that up!" I yelled. But I couldn't bear the mess, and I couldn't allow Steve to bend down with his aching back. Sobbing, I knelt on the rug, weeding mashed fish from the carpet fibers.

Cendra put Steve's anger in perspective. "It's not your fault," she said. "You haven't done anything wrong. I'm sure the food was fine. But he's lost his sense of taste. He's lost his health. He's lost almost everything. He's just plain mad."

As Steve's ire intensified, he sought to excise me from his life. In July, he forbade me to accompany him to Zion. I dropped him off at the airport and he traveled alone, a quick trip, five days of chemotherapy only. At the hospital, he expunged me from the records. He told the social worker that he had "no support system," and that he lived alone.

I stayed with Sally the week Steve was in the hospital, afraid to sleep alone in Steve's apartment in Saline. On the weekend, Sally and I painted the walls of her little house, scrubbed the claw-foot tub, washed windows. The previous tenant, a ninety-five year old man, had been bed-bound and there were long frayed cords attached to pull-chains so he could shut off lights and close doors from his bed. His room became my room, just large enough for a dresser and a single bed, the same one in which the old man had slept. I liked that I had my own room, which I did not have growing up, in college or after, sharing with sisters, roommates, then boyfriends. The room was old-fashioned, with 1950s rose-patterned linoleum and yellowed lace curtains, like my grandmother's. The windows were antique; the hand-blown glass was rippled, which distorted the image outside, a sagging clothesline with a brilliant purple clematis climbing its pole.

The house had a long narrow living room, a stand-in only kitchen, and tiny bathroom. Sally slept in the unfinished attic. She had to pull down a ladder to access her garret hideaway, which blocked the refrigerator door from opening.

On weekdays after work, Sally and I walked over to the wide, slow-moving Huron River, sat on the dock and dangled our feet in the water. Sally set the timer on her camera and photographed us together, she looking off to the east, I to the west, unintentionally opposed, our dresses billowing in the wind. I kept the photo in the glove box of my car so that wherever I traveled, Sally went with me.

On Friday evening, we drove out to Pickerel Pond outside of Ann Arbor, down a rutted two-track to a quiet swimming hole. We unwrapped chèvre and Kalamata olives and a baguette, and uncorked a bottle of wine. As we picnicked, Sally described in exquisite detail the dishes she created at her new job at Zingerman's, a New York style gourmet delicatessen, how delicious they tasted, how quickly they sold.

All week she'd brought home plastic containers for me filled with savory concoctions. Sally and I rarely talked about what was happening with Steve—she appeared uncomfortable if I broached the subject—but feeding me was Sally's way of sustaining me, of showing love.

Sally talked about men she had crushes on: Joe, four years younger, and Rick, who had an on-and-off-again girlfriend. I could see that she had shaken her winter blues and was making a life for herself in Ann Arbor. I was happy for her, and envious. She'd found kindred spirits, artists and musicians and poets, and had been invited to screen entries in a film festival. Several of her paintings were hanging in Del Rio, a funky bar and venue for rising musicians, and she'd enrolled in an art history class, the final course she needed for her bachelor's degree in fine arts.

I laid back in the warm sun with my eyes closed and listened to Sally talk about her life as if she were a character in an off-beat soap opera, her paper on Toulouse-Lautrec, her vivid descriptions of food, her bizarre preposterous dreams, like one in which she saw two babies playing dangerously close to a roof's edge. When she changed one's diaper, she found in it a small frozen chicken.

We laughed, and I told her my dream.

I'm riding my bicycle—a little banana bike with high handle bars and tassels—with Debbie Hartman. Remember her? It's getting darker and darker, the sky and clouds are descending on us, moving toward us, like a storm. Night is coming. We have to get home before dark or we'll freeze. It feels like we might not make it because I can feel the cold already, and so we peddle faster and faster.

Sally was quiet. "Oh," she said, her voice low.

"What?" I said.

"The darkness in the sky. Freezing. It's death." She nearly whispered this.

The translation seemed so obvious after she said it. Even if I didn't dare utter it aloud, subconsciously I couldn't help but fill my mind with metaphors of what was taking place around me each day.

We swam.

The water was tepid in the shallows, minnows swarmed my calves. Waist-deep I dove under, then crawl-stroked toward the center of the pond, watching the sandy bottom turn moldy green then black, my body passing through cold streams from underground springs. In the middle of the pond, I looked up. I could have swam across the tiny pond. I knew I could make it, but I didn't dare. It was something I would have done a year before, but I'd grown fearful of what could happen.

Sally paddled out next to me, floating on a vinyl raft. Someone at work had told her that largemouth bass have giant sharp teeth. They don't bite, I assured her, but she was not taking any chances. I swam back to shore, while Sally drifted all the way to the other side of the pond, lingering there until the sky dimmed, the sun dropping below the tree line. I watched her anxiously in case her raft sank, in case she fell in and got tangled in weeds, ready to rescue her. In theory, I knew how to save a drowning person. Every morning in the summer after eighth grade, I woke at seven for a junior lifesaving class. Fourteen was the youngest age you could enroll, so I was the smallest student. I earned perfect grades on the weekly quizzes, and in practice was able to swim the required distances. I learned the holds, and towed the bodies of my classmates the length of the pool.

The final class was a series of ten practical tests. I executed the releases well (various ways of slipping out of the death-grip of a drowning person). The final test was carrying one of the lifeguards across the pool. I was assigned Rob Sullivan, a cocky, barrel-chested high school senior. I jumped in the water, knees bent and arms akimbo to stay afloat, keeping my eye on Rob, who was histrionically drowning. I maneuvered him into a chin-hold and his legs floated up. I began to side-stroke and was preparing to secure him in a cross-chest carry to tow him ashore, to save his life, but he began to struggle violently and easily broke my chin-hold. "She's not strong enough," he told the instructor, so I failed. This was the first time I'd ever failed a test, failed an entire class, the first time I realized that I *could* fail, that desire plus determination might not be enough.

On Saturday, I picked Steve up at the airport in Detroit. I cooked him dinner, but he didn't touch his food and wouldn't speak to me for most of the night. Finally, he said, "Why are you here?" I sat down next to him on the couch. "I know you don't want to be here," he said. "I don't need your pity."

"I'm here because I love you," I said, exasperated. "Would I put up with all this if I didn't?"

"You're after my money," he said.

I shook my head. "What money? I could earn more working."

"Just get the fuck out," he said softly.

"Fine." I said, calling his bluff. "You're on your own."

I stuffed some clothes into a garbage bag, muffling my sobs, hoping that Steve would capitulate. I dragged the bag out of the bedroom, past Steve on the couch who stubbornly avoided looking at me as he clicked the remote control.

"I'm leaving," I said.

No response.

I slammed the door behind me, and hauled the bag down the stairs bumpety-bump, heaved it into the jeep and drove off. I never reached Sally's house fifteen minutes away. I didn't make it more than two miles down Saline-Ann Arbor Road before I pulled into the parking lot of the Hop-In convenience store, rested my head on the steering wheel and wept. "Bastard!" I yelled. "Why is he doing this? Fucker!" My eyes swelled and nose clogged and lips puffed from biting back frustration. I sat for half an hour, then cleaned myself up and drove back to Saline, where Steve and I spent the night in silence.

Intellectually, I understood Steve's anger. I'd studied Kübler-Ross's theories in my college class, "Death and Dying: Loss as a Part of Life," in which I'd earned an A. In praxis though, I was flunking the course.

Steve's anger reinforced our isolation. People turned away. His parents visited less frequently; they let a month go by without coming to Saline. His friends, the few who'd kept in touch, stopped calling, with the exception of Joey who continued to peddle Dilaudid and deliver money every couple weeks. Steve's cousin Jessica, who'd phoned faithfully every week, no longer called after Steve rebuffed her. She'd asked to borrow his camper for a week. The trailer sat unused in Steve's parents' backyard so the favor seemed reasonable, but it was ill-timed. The week before, Linda had asked to borrow his tent. "They don't give a shit about me," Steve said. "They just want my stuff. They act like I'm dead already."

Bunkered in our apartment day in and day out, we grew cagey. I was angry at Steve for dying, for leaving me. He was mad at me for living, for having left him already. One morning as I cleaned the living room, I saw a notebook on the coffee table and opened it, not out of curiosity but simply to know where it belonged (was it stained glass patterns Steve was sketching or bills to pay?). Inside on blue-lined paper Steve had written his will. I scanned it for just a few seconds before I shut the cover, but long enough to see that he'd divided our possessions among his family: the television to his parents; the bed to his sister; furniture dispersed among them; and to all three children, his cash.

I didn't mention the will to Steve; he hadn't told me he was writing it. But I wrote a letter to my mother and told her that Steve was giving away our stuff, the bed we slept in each night, the couch we sat on, the dresser in which I put my clothes. Or maybe what I found so disturbing was not the dispersal of the material objects but the meaning attached to his designations. We give to those we love, money and objects the currency of affection. It seemed that Steve was willing to take from me without giving in return.

My mother wrote back. *You know you're helping Steve because you love him, and underneath his anger, he loves you.* My mother was right, and her words freed me from my grievance. I put the matter behind me. When Steve said again one day, "You're only here for my money," I looked at him.

"That's ridiculous," I said.

"Oh really?" he replied. "Is that why you complained to your mother about the will?" He must have seen the letter sticking out of my purse and read it while I was asleep.

"What were you doing fishing around in my pocketbook?" I said.

"What were you doing reading my will?"

Steve didn't believe that I'd innocently happened upon his will. He'd never trusted me in our relationship, and he didn't trust me now. I pointed out that he was giving away furniture we'd purchased together, dressers and chairs, the antique tables we'd planned on stripping to raise the oak grain. We'd never gotten around to that project.

"You want everything," Steve said. He sat in his La-Z-Boy. I sat on the couch he'd designated to his sister.

"I don't want everything, Steve, but you're giving away our bed. What am I supposed to sleep on?"

Steve started to cry. "Don't you realize how hard this is for me? You have no idea what it's like to write your will."

We both wept then, and I was awash in a tide of shame.

The most painful heartbreak is not when a lover leaves you, or when someone hurts you, but when by your own actions, ungenerous or cruel or selfish, you break your own heart. I sat on the edge of the coffee table so that I could face Steve. "I'm sorry," I said. "I'm so sorry." He was silent. "I'm not here because I want furniture or money, Steve. I know you don't believe me, but it's true."

In seventh grade, my girlfriends and I wrote our wills once during free period. We divided up our riches: bikes, clothes, jewelry, savings from babysitting. We were capricious and melodramatic. We didn't leave anything to our families. Our allegiance was to our cadre of friends who were more important than anyone else in our small, insulated lives. But that was a game; we couldn't fathom our own demises.

When I turned fifty I wrote a will, only because I had some assets finally, a small retirement fund, a car, a house. In disseminating my possessions, I felt powerful, heady. Money is an aphrodisiac; it seduces. Everyone wants it, few have it. To bestow is a power; to withhold is, too. I found a certain pleasure in the act of writing my will, allowable only because my death remained unimaginable. When Steve said, you don't know what it's like to write your will, he meant, *you don't know what it's like to know you are going to die soon.*

Steve was right that I wanted everything. I wanted Steve to recover completely. I wanted our relationship problems to vanish. I wanted our country home with its solar power and windmill, the fantasy life we'd dreamed of in New York. But I didn't really want Steve's money. I wanted something else in return for my care of him, for my days and nights and weekends, for my love. In return I wanted his love, but that he withheld.

18. The Murmur of Everything Moving

In August, the days were hot and humid. By ten in the morning, the air was inert and scorchy. The heat burned up the grass and broiled the blacktop. I couldn't step onto our deck with bare feet, couldn't touch the wrought iron railing. The intensity of the sun magnified as it passed through our living room windows, turning the apartment into a sauna. I bought a hammock with a metal frame for the veranda, so that at night when the air cooled Steve could recline and study the stars until gravity, the weight of his own body suspended in cloth, began to hurt.

One weekend when Steve was feeling better, we took the kids camping at Higgins Lake in central Michigan, a large, clear-water, sand-bottom lake that stays shallow for so long I never discovered the deep water there. It was like an ocean after time had ceased, caught at low tide forever. Nate balanced his weight on his hands in six inches of water. "Watch me swim," he yelled, crocodiling along. Steve sat in a lawn chair on shore as I swung Lisa around by her arms, skimming the surface of the lake. Sarah practiced handstands, and showed us how long she could hold her breath under water.

At night, we lit a bonfire and roasted marshmallows, waved sparklers in the darkness. Steve was withdrawn and taciturn, but it was more of a sour mood than the bursts of vitriol I'd witnessed lately. Over time, with Cendra's help, I learned to let Steve's fury glide past me like a flock of dark birds. I reminded myself that he was not raging *against* me, but raging *for* his own life.

In the morning while Steve and Nate and Lisa slept, Sarah and I tiptoed down to the lake for a swim. The campground was quiet, the sun just brimming the horizon, streaking the surface of the lake with glassy white-gold light. We were the only two people alive in the world and for the moment we felt entirely free, shivering in the chilly water, dunking under, floating. But soon I worried that Steve would wake up, find us missing and be angry. After twenty minutes, I said, "Come on Sarah, we'd better get back."

Everyone was still sleeping when we returned. Sarah and I could have stayed another half-hour, and I felt sheepish for cutting short her pleasure, for letting her see how anxious and guilty I felt, as if she should feel that way too.

On Sunday morning we packed up to go home. It was only ten a.m., but steamy hot already. "Let's have one more swim before we go," I said.

"No," Steve said. "We're all packed. We're not stopping." He pulled down the dirt road away from our campsite, the trailer neatly tagging along.

"Just a quick dip," I said. "It's so hot." The kids were silent but hopeful. "We won't be long. Come on. They don't get to do this often."

At the last minute, Steve veered into the parking lot at the campground entrance and said, "Make it quick."

The kids and I ran out of the car, changed into bathing suits and splashed around in the lake. We swam as long as I dared, as long as I thought Steve would tolerate. He stood on the shore watching us.

"Come in, Dad," Nate yelled.

"It's warm!" Lisa said.

"Why don't you come in?" I said to Steve. "It's really nice."

He refused. He wouldn't allow himself the carnal delight of immersing his body in cool water on a hot day; he was too angry at his body to indulge it in sensual pleasure.

In that junior lifesaving class so long ago, I learned how to approach a drowning person. If the victim's head was still above water, you must nose-dive a few feet in front of him, grab his ankles, and turn his body away from you. If you swim directly up to the flailing victim, in his panic he will clutch onto you, try to climb you, push you under. In your panic, you do the same and entwined, united, two as one, you sink to the bottom. Separated, at least one of you might survive.

In late August, Steve announced that he would travel to Zion alone, and for once I didn't argue. On this trip, bone scans revealed that his cancer had further metastasized. Dr. Sanchez switched Steve's chemotherapy to Velban, a more toxic drug that made Steve feel hot and sick to his stomach. Then the doctor changed Steve's prognosis from "in control" to "guarded."

At home, Steve was weaker than ever. All he wanted was peace and quiet, but we lived a block up from Route 12, a four lane highway that spanned Michigan from Detroit in the eastern corner of the state all the way west to Indiana. Our apartment was in a neighborhood of closely-situated houses, above a family with two boys. Besides cars backfiring and revving, and trucks and lawn mowers rumbling, the landlord's oldest son blasted rock music downstairs when his parents weren't home.

On Steve's first Saturday back, a dozen ten-year-old boys, friends of our landlord's younger son, screamed and yelled and ran around the yard. It was too hot to close the windows and we didn't have an air conditioner. The bass from their stereo thumped up through the floor. I walked downstairs and knocked on the front door. "Is there any way you can turn the music down? Steve's not feeling well."

"This is a birthday party," Melissa said. "What do you expect?"

"It's really loud," I said. "Can you turn it down a little?"

"This is my son's birthday!" she said "You shouldn't even be living here. He's sick, he should be home. Why don't you go home," she said, then closed the door.

"She won't turn it down," I told Steve. I soaked a washcloth in cold water and draped it on his forehead. "It won't last much longer. Let me run to the drug store and buy earplugs. I'll get you some ginger ale."

Later that evening from our living room window Steve and I saw Joey turn into the block and park his car across the street. We waited to hear the rattle of the screen door, but it never came. After several minutes we walked out on the veranda, where we found Joey slumped in a lawn chair, his eyes shut as if he were sleeping. "Hey Joe," Steve said, stepping out onto the deck in his black and white checked bathrobe, the deck's tar-paper surface still warm from the hot day.

Joey was woozy and drugged, clearly distraught.

"What's the matter?" Steve asked, sitting in a folding lawn chair. I sat on the step to the kitchen door.

"Phil got killed in a motorcycle accident," Joey said, slurring.

Steve and I were silent. There was nothing we could say. We couldn't even mourn Phil. We hadn't known him really, hadn't liked him, and even if we had, we couldn't allow the concept of grief too near. We kept it distant and strange, did not let it enter our house.

"Seems like everyone around me is dying," Joey said.

I appreciated Joey's impropriety. Nobody else, not Steve, not I articulated the truth so plainly. The three of us sat quietly listening to the steady music of the cars and trucks speeding by on Route 12, so close to our apartment, traveling so fast. Nights like this—the balmy air, the sound of traffic—made me feel as if I could be anywhere, California, Indiana, it was all the same. I felt a placelessness, a sense that it didn't matter where on earth I was, that it would be this way always; that everywhere there were people sitting, motors thrumming, houses and porches and trees.

Sitting on the veranda with Steve and Joey, I felt time passing, *felt* it in my body like a shiver, the sun setting, the temperature dropping. A man across the street—a neighbor Steve and I had never met or spoken to, a man who was a stranger to us, which saddened me because now it was too late to get to know the neighbors, to live the way we should have—carefully pulled on garden gloves to mow his lawn, then plucked rocks out of the grass and chucked them into the street.

The landlord's son and his friends, dressed in fatigues, pretended the rocks were grenades and dove for the ground. They ran from tree to tree for cover, screaming, "badadadadada… got ya," pitching themselves to the lawn, clutching their chests. They played war every day after school, after dinner, on weekends, with black grease paint smudged under their eyes, wielding authentic looking automatic weapons. I wondered if they would ever tire of the game, of killing and dying over and over.

A row of starlings perched on the telephone line looked like eighth notes on a staff, no melody but a rapid single note struck again and again. Joey formed his index finger into a pistol, aimed at the birds. Pshu, pshu. He stood up, pulled a clump of damp twenties out of his pocket, dropped it on the small metal table. "I gotta go," he said.

Steve and I watched him stagger down the stairs, start his car, and turn onto Route 12, his engine blending with the murmur of everything moving.

Summer broke. September was cool and pretty. The supple star-shaped leaves of the sugar maples bled into shiny brown-red. The elms and ashes flared yellow and orange. I've always liked September, the back-to-school season, boys and girls in new shoes, fresh haircuts, grown taller. Days were structured again. Everyone, even children, had something important to attend. My mother told me once that of her seven children, I was the only one who cried on the first day of school for many years. What did I dread? What loss did I sense? I loved school and in those elementary years was an excellent student. Maybe I cried for the loss of the capaciousness of summer, hours passed immersed in books, the wildness of days spent exploring woods and swamps, climbing trees. Maybe each fall I sensed the passing of time. Time gone, vanished so quickly; that in itself was mournful.

That autumn, Steve's anger, like a monsoon season, ended. And though each day was easier because of his calm—he no longer ordered me to leave weekly, he no longer complained about the food I cooked—I mourned the loss of his fury. His anger had embodied his will to live.

October. Leaves fell in long dillydallying descents, accumulating quickly on the sidewalks. Days shortened, though it seemed more obvious that autumn, the cycles and stages, continuity dramatized, or at least the ending of things. I wrote in my journal: *Some nice memories of Steve...* followed by a long list of reminiscences, as if he were gone already.

When I'd taken the drawing class the year before Steve fell ill, we'd progressed from self-portraiture to figure drawing. I'd started sketching Steve one day as he sat in his La-Z-Boy recliner, but when he noticed, he refused to pose. He did not want to be captured by my charcoals, perhaps concerned how I'd render him. Instead I drew the chair, spending hours replicating each tiny crochet loop Grandma Nettie had stitched in the doily draped over its back. In the end, my portrait of Steve did not include him, though it *was* him. Illustrating the chair's angles and textures, the slight depression in the seat cushion as if Steve had just risen from the chair, created a tension, an aliveness to the sketch that, despite being uninhabited, contained a body in the form of an implication, a memory, as if Steve had just gotten up to get a drink from the fridge. But perhaps the drawing was an augury: a portrait of absence.

When Steve recovered from chemotherapy that month, we drove north for a weekend to The Sands Motel near the tip of Michigan's

Lower Peninsula, where the landscape pushed up into small hills. Our room had a luxurious king-size bed in which we both slept so soundly and deeply that we asked the hotel manager the brand of the mattress, as if it were a magic bed. We vowed to buy one when we returned home, as if it had been a bed all along that we lacked, that could deliver the relief we craved.

At night we soaked our bodies in the outdoor spa; the steaming moil of water soothed Steve's aches. That night in the hot tub—gazing at the veil of the Milky Way, warm swirling water soothing Steve's aches—was the single moment of physical pleasure for Steve in the nine months since he was diagnosed.

On Saturday, we drove out to a nearby livery, signed a liability waiver, and with a handful of other tourists, mounted slow, seasoned horses for a guided amble through the woods. I'd only been horseback riding once before and so I gripped the reigns tightly and nervously. Steve and I were the last plodding riders. "Hold back," he said, stopping in the path.

"Why?" I asked. What was he planning, an escape? A ride off into the wilderness, into a new scene, a new life?

"So we can gallop."

We waited for the group to advance well ahead of us, the space across a meadow widening. I was frightened as I kicked the horse's flank and it charged ahead, but my fear was coupled with the thrill of our hijack, the transgressive pleasure, speed and recklessness. At least that's how I felt, out of control. Steve was fully in charge. It was gratifying to see him relaxed and in command, harnessing the might of the horse's powerful body.

On our way back to the stables we encountered another group of riders. "Head over this way," our guide said, leading us off the trail, past a split rail fence. Suddenly my horse whinnied and reared on her hindquarters, boxed the air with her forelegs. I clamped my thighs and held on. A stallion thundered up to the fence a few feet away and brayed and paced and snorted. I could see his large menacing yellow teeth. I kicked my horse in the gut and she bolted a few hundred yards. My heart punched lubb dupp lubb dupp, galloping even after my mare had stopped and was quietly munching grass. The leader sidled up next to me. "Are you alright?" she asked. "I guess your mare is in heat. Good thing the stallion didn't jump the fence."

Good thing. I was still trembling as I dismounted at the stable and Steve and I drove away. Steve comforted me, but we were on the verge of giggling, filled with nervous energy, exhilarated, thrilled to be shook up, our blood pumping, from the near escape from danger. We'd survived calamity.

That week at work, on a chilly sunless day, a typical fall day in Michigan, sometime in the afternoon I became nearly paralyzed sitting at my desk, stunned and slow like a winter bee. My mind froze. I couldn't think and I couldn't catch my breath, as if I'd just ascended a steep hill. My body tingled yet felt weighted, like the force of gravity had doubled. What had I just been working on? The typescript on the page blurred. I had to do something. I began to rubberstamp envelopes. Steady, simple, mindless. But the feeling persisted. I walked upstairs to the storage room where it was dark and stood among the stacks of cartons. I stayed there for some length of time; I couldn't gauge how long, probably no more than fifteen minutes but everything had gelled, thickened, and so it felt longer. I inhaled slowly and deeply and finally the fog in my mind dissipated.

A panic attack. I remembered the description from my Abnormal Psychology class in college. How strange, I mused. Out of the blue. I still didn't register the cause behind the attack. My body knew to panic, knew that something awful loomed even if I didn't consciously register the closeness of death. The dailiness of Steve's dying disguised its intensity. Death had become quotidian.

I returned to my desk, picked up where I'd left off: writing a press release.

In November, Steve traveled to Zion for another round of Velban. His response to the medication, according to Dr. Sanchez, was "excellent," and so the dose was increased. Dr. Sanchez and Dr. Melijor remained optimistic about Velban, and for their hope I was grateful and slightly astonished. They kept trying valiantly to save Steve as if they cared about him, as if he wasn't just one of millions of cancer patients in the world, as if he were a concert pianist or a brilliant mathematician instead of an ordinary man, an electrician, a father.

Steve grew more optimistic about his future. When the social worker queried him about his support system, he answered, "My girlfriend." I was back in the picture. But the Velban was harsh. It gave Steve painful stomach cramps—short sharp kicks—and his white blood cell count sank to its lowest level. He was so nauseated that he couldn't hold down Ensure, the protein drink for the elderly. His hands and feet were numb, and now they kicked out involuntarily while he was awake, not just when he slept. Chemotherapy is so crude a treatment, like trying to remove a splinter with an axe.

At home, Steve was helpless. I couldn't get him to eat anything for days, and he lost eight more pounds. He leaned heavily on me when he needed to use the bathroom, draping his dead-weight arm around my shoulder, surprisingly dense and heavy for someone who appeared so thin and bird-boned. I felt the weight of his body like never before, and I felt his absence. He was so ponderously fatigued, as if he could never get enough sleep. He woke from sleeping exhausted, slept more, woke again and was immediately tired. He slept so many hours of every day and night as if he'd gone into hibernation, like Rip Van Winkle with his long white beard twenty years overgrown. My father had read that story to me at bedtime when I was a girl, and I remember feeling anxious that I might fall asleep and never wake up.

Steve called me at work one day, the first time he'd done so in ten months of illness.

"I just threw up," he said quietly. "It's all over the bathroom floor."

"Don't worry about it," I said. "Go lay down. I'll be right home."

"I have to leave," I told Phyllis. "Steve's really sick."

"Are you coming back?" she asked.

"Tomorrow," I said.

November delivered Michigan's usual gray pallor. It was cold and barren, but I welcomed this weather. I didn't feel glum about being stuck inside. Instead I relished being sequestered in the apartment, warm and cozy with Grandma Nettie's afghan spread over Steve lying back on the couch, his heavy legs draped across my lap as we watched television.

An article I'd written months before about Phyllis and her business was finally being published. "*Executive Female* is running the profile on you," I told her.

"*Executive Female?*" she said. "Only shrews read that."

"My sister reads it," I said. My oldest sister, Susan, was earning her M.B.A. at night, working full-time during the day. After that I began to peruse the employment section in the paper. In late November, the director of The Nature Conservancy, a nonprofit environmental group, called me to arrange a job interview for the Director of Development position. I was elated. I've considered myself an environmentalist since I was ten, when I helped clean up roadside trash on the very first Earth Day in 1970. In seventh grade, for my science report on pollution, my father drove me into Boston to photograph smokestacks, and I'd taken snapshots of the car dump in the woods behind my house.

Before the interview, Cendra advised me to be honest about Steve's situation. She gave me words to say if I thought I was close to being hired. *I'm taking care of my boyfriend who's dying of cancer, so I won't be able to start until after January.* I rehearsed. I read library books on fund raising. I drew a chart of possible ways to raise money. I tried to make my hair comply to some conventional style with a handful of bobby pins. I wore a pink knit vest over a white blouse, a striped linen skirt that I bought at the Salvation Army store: quality fabric, even if used.

I sat at the end of a long table in a conference room at a hotel in Lansing, an hour and a half from Saline. Four men in suits stared at me. One was the publisher of a chain of newspapers in Michigan. He looked like an owl with his bushy, peaked eyebrows and hooked nose. A tall, thin aristocratic man was a vice president of Ford Motor Company. The third man, balding and kindly-looking, was the attorney for Michigan's governor. They were members of The Nature Conservancy's Board of Directors. The executive director, Tom, was a gregarious sort, handsome in an unkempt way, with recessed blue eyes set close together, and a nose that surely had been broken. He shook my hand vigorously and grinned a toothy smile.

"Tell us about yourself," Tom said, and leaned back, folding his arms across his chest, which I couldn't help notice was one of those strange concave ones.

I didn't know where to start, as dislocated in the world as I felt. I was afraid that if I pulled one thread of my carefully tucked-in countenance, I'd unravel, and that's what happened. I babbled. I heard myself saying something about my family, brothers and sisters, liberal politics. It sounded wrong amidst these suited executives, but I couldn't control my words, couldn't define myself with a few bold strokes. I perspired, and felt a curl of hair loosening at my brow, wriggling out of its clip.

Tom asked, "What would you do as Director of Development?"

I pulled out my chart and noticed slight approving nods. I began to relax and speak more coherently, even though the curl had sprung loose;

I could see its shadow. I felt like the girl with the curl in the middle of her forehead. *When she's good, she's very very good. When she's bad, she's very very bad.* I struggled to control a tremor in my chest that I feared would manifest as hysterical giggling or sobbing.

At the end of the interview, Tom told me that I was one of four final candidates.

"If you were hired," he asked, "when could you start?"

I silently thanked Cendra for my stock line, which I spoke without emotion. "I'm taking care of my boyfriend who's dying of cancer, so I won't be able to start until after January."

"Pardon me if this sounds inappropriate," Tom asked, "but how long do you expect him to live?"

His question caught me off-guard. Cendra hadn't scripted this one. "He probably won't make it to next year," I said.

The men thanked me, and we shook hands.

Afterward, speeding along the highway toward home, toward Steve all alone in that drab apartment day after day, sleeping, watching television, his life slowly ebbing, I replayed Cendra's words, my words, in my mind, steering with one hand as I pulled bobby pins out of my hair, coming unwound then, the road in front of me blurring as the tears came.

In December, Steve was scheduled to return to Zion, but he didn't want to ruin Christmas so he delayed booking a flight. I saw an advertisement on television for a home spa, and I decided that I must obtain one for Steve, this machine that would transform our bathtub into a whirlpool, like the one at the Sands Motel. I searched department stores in Ann Arbor and Ypsilanti for the spa, but the spa was the hot item that year and every place was sold out. *I have to get the spa.* The spa would bring Steve many hours of pure comfort; his pain would melt away in the warm, bubbling waters of our own home spa.

I called my sisters and mother and asked them to look for the spa in Massachusetts and New York. My mother eventually found one and shipped it in time for Christmas, and Steve, as hopeful as I was, tried the spa right after the holiday. I ran a bath and placed the plastic base at the bottom of the tub. The base was like a small surfboard, thick and hard, with hundreds of tiny holes, and a vacuum cleaner-type hose which snaked over the edge of the tub and connected to a helmet-shaped motor set on our tile floor. The tub filled with four inches of hot water, and then the faucet ran cold. Steve stepped gingerly into the tub and arranged his body over the plastic base. I turned the motor on and it sounded like we were running a chainsaw in the bathroom. I folded a towel under the motor to muffle the sound.

"How does it feel?" I asked Steve.

"It's freezing," he said, half-laughing, his gangly legs folded awkwardly, pencil-thin arms hanging over the edge of the bathtub. He lasted another minute before he started shivering and I helped him out of the tub.

"Doesn't it work?" I asked.

"Try it," he said.

He didn't want to appear ungrateful. The spa cost over a hundred dollars, half of my weekly salary then, and he knew the trouble I'd had finding one. I'd told him of the all-out search, perhaps to heighten his appreciation of the gift, or perhaps because that small adventure was of exaggerated importance in our life so devoid of fulfilling events—we rarely did anything or went anywhere.

Steve put on his robe as I immersed myself in the tub. The water was frigid, and I realized that the motor sucked in the cold air from the bathroom and compressed it through the tiny holes in the base, which created effervescence, like lying in a tub of ginger ale, but which quickly and effectively cooled the shallow water. With the annoying rumble of the motor and the awkward discomfort of lying on the hard plastic mat, I realized the spa was utterly useless: a poor design.

My mother and everyone else I'd assigned to search for the spa called to inquire about Steve's reaction. When I felt helpless to relieve Steve's pain, I grasped onto any possible balm and built it into more than it could ever promise. That's what hope does: inflates. All that I longed to give Steve—comfort, health, pleasure—was brought to bear onto an object. So when the thing failed, a thing which was after all nothing more than plastic extruded from a mold, there was an emotional symmetry: the disappointment was as amplified as the hope had been.

19. Brompton's Cocktail

Late January, 1987. About a year since Steve was first diagnosed with cancer, a third of our relationship. Is it apt to say that time flew? It seems that it did, probably because we did not think we'd make it that far. That was how we survived: gaze to the ground, plodding ahead, taking small footsteps. That was how time rushed past, by averting our eyes from the clock, the calendar, ignoring what lay ahead, parsing time into manageable increments: this minute, this hour, this day.

That January, Dr. Sanchez called. "I'm not coming back," I heard Steve say. He told the doctor that he might try the Bahamas clinic, but I knew he was putting off Dr. Sanchez, who'd remained true to his first promise: *we don't give up that easily.* I was surprised. Steve hadn't told me about his decision to end treatment. Maybe it wasn't a decision at all, just an impulsive response. Or perhaps it was inertia. Two months had passed since he'd traveled to Zion; a body at rest stays at rest.

"Why aren't you going back?" I asked.

"I feel worse from the treatment. It's not worth it," Steve said, without specifying the first *it*: the beating of his heart, waking and sleeping and eating each day; thinking, laughing, talking, loving. *It* was his life.

"There are other things they can try. We didn't ask about interferon. You could try hyperthermia again."

"What the use?" Steve said. "We're never going to get married."

I was taken aback. "That's not true," I said. "We'll get married. We can work out our problems. Look at what we've been through."

"No," Steve said. "I don't think so."

I let the discussion rest, figuring that I'd convince him over time. He wrote me a letter soon after.

Cheer up, Mo. I guess I'd be going crazy if I were in your place, knowing that any time you could die, never before feeling love like I have with you. I don't want to die, but what do I have to live for? At first I thought we could have a happy life together, buy a house, get married, spend more time with the kids. But I don't think this will ever happen.

I tried to reassure Steve. "We will get married," I said. "We will."

But I could not convince him that a rosy, blissful wedded life waited for us just beyond the cancer treatment, especially when only six months prior I'd refused to move back in with him, on paper at least.

Steve's decision not to return to Zion marked his acknowledgment of the inevitable outcome of his illness: the end of his life, though it was less a discernible acceptance than a gradual letting-go of anger, fear, denial. In acknowledging death, Steve began to live again, to resume some of the pleasures he'd suspended. He took up smoking with a vengeance, lighting a fresh cigarette with the ember of the one before it. We abandoned the health food diet and I cooked Steve's favorite foods, apple crisp and roast Cornish game hens with potatoes and gravy, fat and sugar and refined white flour and additives and chemical ingredients, known carcinogens.

We gorged. Or at least I did. I baked and cooked to satisfy Steve's cravings. If he wanted a Rice Krispy treat, I made a batch. He'd eat one square—his appetite was still poor—and I'd eat the rest of the pan, unable to stop myself. When he wanted another, I'd make a second pan, cut him a square, and eat the remainder, standing in the kitchen, shoving gobs of batter into my mouth. I craved cookies and desserts, sugar a quick fix to satisfy some hunger, some need beyond hunger. I gained pounds as Steve shed weight.

Steve worked on stained glass, and we watched even more movies, two and three a day, six or seven on weekends. We joked and snuggled on the couch, and kissed a little. We stopped arguing completely, abruptly. Arguing was staking a claim for the future, to change each other, to alter an outcome. Continuing to fight was continuing to hang on to the idea of a future. Once we let go of denial, we forfeited our grievances.

We became lovers again, not because we were able to make love—Steve was too weak, and sick, and still suffered burning in his urethra—but because we fell in love again, like in New York but different, a mature love, less a cycle of thrilling fits of passion focused around our lusty bodies, less a desire to possess each other, more like a slow-burning bed of coals, warmth and intimacy, like people who'd been married for fifty years. That's how I saw us, an old retired couple, slow-moving, with nothing much to do, time on our hands, but then again, not really, not much.

Dr. Sanchez mailed Steve a letter stating his condition so that a Michigan physician could prescribe narcotics. I called a doctor in Saline whose office was only two blocks from our apartment, and when I explained Steve's situation, he generously offered to make a house call. Dr. Thorton was in his late thirties, with longish hair for a professional, and casual attire, khakis and a dress shirt. He knocked on the door and walked into our living room with his black bag, and introduced himself to Steve. They shook hands. Dr. Thorton bent over to speak to Steve sitting in his La-Z-Boy. "What are you taking now?" he asked.

Steve pointed to the bottles of morphine and Dilaudid on the coffee table.

Dr. Thorton picked them up and read the labels. "How are you feeling?"

Steve started to cry, one of the few times I'd witnessed him crying in the year he'd been ill. "My back hurts so much," Steve said. "Can you give me something stronger?"

"There's really nothing stronger than these," Dr. Thorton said.

"Can you prescribe a Brompton's cocktail?" I asked. I'd read that this was the most potent painkiller—a highball of morphine and cocaine.

"I can't prescribe a Brompton's cocktail," Dr. Thorton said sharply. "You won't find anyone around here who will. I'm sorry." He stood upright. "There's nothing I can do."

He hadn't opened his medical bag, hadn't sat on our couch. He strode quickly out of our apartment, the screen door slamming behind him.

A day later, Steve received a letter from Dr. Thorton stating that he couldn't prescribe narcotics because, in his professional opinion, Steve was addicted to the drugs.

"Well no shit," Steve said. "Of course I'm addicted, but I'm not an *addict*."

We began to worry. Steve had two days of pain medication left, and no prescription. I called Cendra and she called her friend, Ingrid, who operated a hospice and home nursing service in Ann Arbor. Ingrid called a doctor who agreed to prescribe medication for three days, enough to last the weekend until Steve could come in for an appointment. We breathed a sigh of relief, until I learned that the Saline pharmacy didn't stock Dilaudid. I called drug stores listed in the phone book. St. Joseph's Hospital pharmacy in Ypsilanti was the only place that carried the medication. I drove there, but the pharmacist wouldn't fill the prescription because it wasn't written by a doctor affiliated with the hospital. That was our last option, and I strained to keep my emotions in check.

"This man is running out of medication," I said to the pharmacist. "He'll be in pain."

"We can't break the rules," he replied.

"You don't understand," I said. "He's dying of cancer." My voice quivered and rose in pitch. People waiting for their prescriptions pretended not to stare at me.

"I'm sorry," the pharmacist said, and for a second I felt as if I might leap over the counter and choke him. So many people who were sorry they couldn't help, so many powerless, sorry people. I called Ingrid's agency, but she was not there. The nurse who answered suggested the name of a doctor, and cheerfully recited his number.

"Can you call?" I asked. Didn't she understand that I was at a pay phone in the lobby of a hospital? That I was desperate and powerless and scared, unable now to contain the surge of tears. She said she'd page Ingrid and I should call her back in fifteen minutes. I stood outside in the cold air, in front of the entrance to St. Joseph's Hospital, a year after Steve was first admitted there, back where we started, begging for help.

The hospice agency couldn't find a doctor affiliated with St. Joseph's who would prescribe narcotics without examining Steve, and he couldn't get an appointment for a few days. One doctor agreed to prescribe Tylenol 3. Ingrid had a bottle of liquid morphine, which the family of a patient who'd recently died donated to her agency, and this held us over until we found a doctor willing to examine Steve's records and write a bottomless prescription for narcotics.

20. The Price is Right

Inside every patient there's a poet trying to get out.
Anatole Broyard

While I dressed for work in the mornings, Steve ate breakfast, Frosted Mini-Wheats. He carried the box into the living room, along with a bowl of milk he set on the coffee table. He plunked one square of cereal into the bowl, waited for it to reach the right degree of saturation, not too soggy, and ate it in one slurpy mouthful. Then he'd soak another biscuit. He had the time for this, to endeavor for the perfect consistency with each bite of cereal. I left him in the middle of this ritual each morning.

One day, I came home from work to find that Steve had written a poem. The poem was simple, rhyming, but I found his effort courageous: the desire for form and order, the impulse toward poetry to seek understanding for what was impossible to fathom. Poems apply intellect to emotion, perhaps diffusing despair. I only know that Steve felt pleasure and a small measure of pride in his poem.

The second line of Steve's poem was, *I have six months till I die.* How did he know? And the last line surprised me: *God is always with you.* Neither Steve nor I prayed aloud, said grace, or attended Mass. Perhaps his mother had influenced him after all. From the beginning, she'd sent religious cards weekly, enclosing pages she'd torn out of the Bible, underscoring passages in florescent yellow marker like I did in college textbooks. Psalm 55:22: "Cast thy burden upon the Lord and he shall sustain thee." She wrote to Steve, urging him to see their pastor. *The only way you will find peace is to get yourself into a right relationship with God. You may not feel your illness is a blessing, but in one way it is. You have time to get right with God.* I never understood Steve's parents' faith in god; he certainly hadn't helped much here on earth. Nor could I see Steve's illness as a blessing; it was almost an insult, I thought, to view it that way. His death would not be a blessing for his young children.

About a year after Steve's diagnosis, in one of her weekly letters Louise enclosed a two-inch square of cornflower-blue fabric cut with pinking shears. The swatch had been anointed and blessed by a faith healer. Steve was to place the cloth on his chest, according to her hand-written instructions, and recite passages from the Bible, including John 3:16: "God loved the world so much that he gave his only Son, that anyone who has faith in him may not die but have eternal life." Steve and I felt silly as I placed the cloth on Steve's chest and he recited the verse, as if we were clicking the heels of ruby slippers. But there was no harm in trying.

A couple weeks later, Steve's mother called to say that the faith healer was coming to Detroit, so on a cold winter night Steve and I drove to Cobo Hall, a huge complex with four levels, and a parking garage underground. We parked and in the lobby walked past the looming statue of Joe Louis, twenty-four feet tall, posed in fight stance, ready to throw a punch. Steve had loved the sport of boxing, loved sparring with a heavy bag. I never understood the appeal of watching men punch each other; I couldn't stomach the violence.

Steve and I found our way to the top level of a huge auditorium, stadium seats cascading below us. The cement floor vibrated beneath our feet as thousands of people stomped and clapped, singing, "Mine eyes have seen the glory of the coming of the Lord." We surveyed the scene around us: paralyzed veterans in wheelchairs, old women with canes, cerebral palsy children limp in their father's arms. I saw people like Steve, wracked by disease. A man hawked sodas, like at a ball game, which seemed strange, as if there should be no thirst here. Down on the floor of the hall were designates, a squadron of fifty or so men and women in ankle-length red robes. The preacher on stage wore a business suit, and was surrounded by palm trees and leafy tropical plants, the same setup as the "No Money Down" real estate seminar Steve and I had attended in that same auditorium two years before.

The preacher shouted into the microphone for anyone who wanted to be healed to come down to the floor, like Bob Barker on *The Price is Right*. Streams of people merged into the aisles and pushed down the steps to receive a gift from the Lord, greedy for salvation and healing. Steve and I joined the swell. On the main floor, women were crying and speaking in tongues, garbled and guttural, writhing in the aisles.

We watched for some time, then Steve shuffled forward to take his place in line. I sat in a fold-up chair at the edge of the crowd and watched the healer, a matronly-looking woman, place her hands on Steve's throat as if she were going to throttle him. She asked him to close his eyes and repeat her words while she massaged the back of his neck.

A minute later she pushed lightly on Steve's chest and he fell back a step, and opened his eyes. He walked over to me.

"How do you feel?" I asked.

"The same," he said. His voice was soft, like cotton.

"Maybe it takes a while," I offered.

"That's what the lady said, I'll feel better in a few days."

Steve decided to wander around to watch others being healed.

"I'll be right here," I promised.

A middle-aged man in a red robe approached me, asked if I'd been healed.

"I'm not sick," I said.

"You must have something that bothers you." He seemed giddy, and I was curious.

"I get neck aches now and then."

"Stand up," he commanded and I obeyed. I wanted him to dispel my doubt, to make a believer of me. He wrapped his hands around my neck and his fingers strayed to the dip behind my earlobes, the place where I would dab perfume if I wore it. He applied pressure, which didn't hurt, but I knew my equilibrium was centered there, in the Eustachian tubes. The designate spoke but I couldn't concentrate. His foul breath blew warmly in my face like a current. He pressed against my sternum. "You will have no more problems with your neck," he said, then turned to heal someone else.

Steve returned. "I've been healed," I said.

"Let's get the fuck out of here," he replied.

Handicapped people who came in wheelchairs, left in wheelchairs. Steve and I wended our way through the labyrinth of hallways to the parking garage below-ground. In another auditorium at Cobo Hall an Ozzy Osborne concert had just ended. Drunk and stoned teenagers in black leather jackets, studded dog collars, and tee-shirts featuring Ozzy baring bloody canines merged with the flow of people from the faith healing. Ten years before, in 1977, I was one of those teenagers, seeing Ozzy with the Black Sabbath band at the Orpheum Theater in Boston, dry ice smoke curling onto the stage as Ozzy emerged squirting a huge penis-shaped water gun, singing, "My name is Lucifer, please take my hand."

Nobody moved. A car had broken down in the only lane out of the parking garage, trapping us all in a cement cell, all of us slowly asphyxiating. The Ozzy Osborne fans began to yell and jump on car roofs, the faith-healer people rolled up their windows and locked their doors. One leather-clad Ozzy fan leered into our passenger window, saw Steve, pale, gaunt, death-kissed, and backed away. Eventually, the teenagers grew bored and tired of protesting, or perhaps they succumbed to carbon monoxide sleepiness. After forty-five minutes, the disabled car was removed and we were freed. Gone, too, was our foolish hope.

21. Self-deliverance

My soul is weary of my life.
Job 10:4

Steve's illness was so intense, so all-consuming that the perimeter of the world closed in around us. Our focus was solely on each other, as it had been in New York when we'd fallen in love. Over time, we navigated an increasingly compressed sphere, a tight orbit between Saline and Zion. When Steve stopped treatment, the orbit was constricted further, shutting Steve away from the external world altogether, confining him to the rooms of our apartment: living room, bathroom, bedroom.

In mid-May, Steve suffered a spell of nausea stemming from severe constipation, a side effect of the morphine. I called Ingrid's hospice service and the nurse suggested a regular regimen of enemas, suppositories, and oral flushes. After two weeks, Steve's vomiting subsided, but he'd taken a step down in health—he was incrementally less mobile, slept just a little longer each day—and this decline became the new standard.

Then his bone pain worsened.

The hospice nurse implanted a needle into Steve's thigh, the only place on his body where he had pinchable flesh. The syringe and tubing were connected to a morphine drip, a portable pump the size of a paperback, which delivered narcotics into Steve's bloodstream. The pump was programmed to allow for one extra dose per hour above the regularly infusing dose, which I could release by pushing a button.

The syringe had to be refilled every four hours, which meant that after loading a fresh supply into the pump at midnight, I'd set the alarm for four a.m. to refill it, and rose at eight in morning to begin the cycle again. Within days, I grew sleep deprived, like a new mother with nightly feedings, weepy, cranky, and emotionally raw.

One afternoon, I asked Steve, "Are you afraid to die?"

"No," he said. "I'm just afraid of more pain."

It was at this time, under these conditions that Steve began to talk about ending his life. "I just want this to be over," he said one day when his back ached terribly. Steve had been hanging on to his tenuous health for nearly a year and a half. He was exhausted, and so he opened the door to the idea of dying. Kübler-Ross called this acceptance, but that wasn't the right word. Acceptance implied agreement or even willingness. Resignation or surrender was a more apt term.

Yet there was defiance in Steve's admission of defeat: if cancer was to be Steve's fate, at least he would trump the gods by choosing the time and manner of his death. "I should just kill myself," he said one night.

After he mentioned this several more times, I took his comment literally

"If that's what you want to do, I'll help you," I said. I contacted the Hemlock Society and they sent instructions for ending one's life. Their booklet referred to suicide as "Self-Deliverance," as if you were packing up your body and shipping the parcel via UPS. To where, though? Maybe one of those self-storage units that seemed to be everywhere.

The technique the Society recommended was called Final Exit, like a stage direction in theater. The first step was to carefully calculate the combination of pills to aid sleep, and an anti-emetic so you wouldn't vomit. Then you placed a plastic bag loosely over your head; not tightly or you'd feel like you were suffocating and want to remove it. They recommended an oven bag, the kind you use to roast a Thanksgiving turkey: long enough, wide enough, light weight. Wearing a dust mask, they noted, would prevent you from sucking the plastic bag into your mouth and nose. A cheap paper type was good enough, like the kind Steve used when he ground stained-glass pieces; the fine whitish glass dust coated his work area. The Hemlock Society suggested a cocktail to help the absorption of drugs, vodka, whiskey or brandy, like a nightcap. If the instructions were followed correctly, death ensued thirty minutes after the onset of sleep.

I consulted Cendra about Steve committing suicide.

"Does he have a gun?" she asked.

Steve hunted, like all the men in his family, and I knew he kept a pistol in the nightstand drawer, which I'd shot once before, with Steve and his sister and her husband shortly after I'd moved to Michigan. We aimed at targets across a field, shooting for sport, for entertainment, but it wasn't something I enjoyed and I never went again.

"Remove the gun," Cendra said. "Get it out of the apartment as soon as possible."

"Why?" I asked. "If Steve wants to end his life, shouldn't he be able to?"

"Of course," she said. "But I'm thinking of you. If you come home and find that mess, you'll be devastated."

One day while Steve slept, I quietly opened the drawer of the nightstand and lifted his pistol; the gun was heavier than I remembered. I placed it in a shoe box for Steve's parents to take away, glad to have it banished from our home.

Louise contacted a Lutheran minister in Saline who began to visit Steve regularly. Pastor Scanlon, a soft-spoken, solicitous young man carried a carved teak box containing holy water to bless Steve, and communion wafers, which he placed on Steve's tongue.

"Would you like communion?" he asked me one day.

I declined. I hadn't received communion in over a decade, since I'd made my confirmation in ninth grade, nor had I kneeled in a confessional booth. I didn't feel holy or worthy, and I'd never really believed in the Christian god, who existed in my mind as a cartoonish figure, a white man with a hazy corona of yellow, wearing a powder blue gown, images from my childhood catechism. "Don't blame this on God," Steve said to me one day. But my beliefs, my faith or lack of it, didn't matter. Pastor Scanlon was there for Steve, and he comforted and soothed Steve in a way that nobody else could.

After a few weeks of Pastor Scanlon's ministrations, Steve changed his mind about suicide. He ceased to mention it, and when I asked him if he was still thinking about it, he said no, because it was forbidden in the Bible. Instead, he decided to spend his last days in the company of his pain because, according to Christianity, suicide was a sin (thou shalt not kill, even yourself). The souls of those who committed suicide could not enter heaven, instead dwelling forever in limbo, which I envisioned from Sunday school as a hoary netherworld just under the earth's crust, not deep enough for the fiery pits of hell, more like a walk-out basement, or the earth-berm home Steve had once imagined building. Pope Benedict would dismiss the concept of limbo twenty year later, but before that, for Steve, spiritual solace was worth bodily suffering.

While Steve was preparing to die, I was searching for a new job. Phyllis fired Monica after she discovered that instead of processing orders, she'd stuffed them in the bottom of a drawer underneath boxes of crackers and dried soups, none of which Monica claimed when she left. Within days, Phyllis hired Stacy, an acquaintance from her country club. With five employees, Phyllis arranged to offer health insurance and so one day an agent met with the staff. We gathered around a conference table and he asked each of us how much we earned. Rebecca and Maggie and Greta and I were shocked to hear that Stacy's salary was higher than all of ours who'd been employed longer, whose positions were purportedly higher than Stacy's in the tiny hierarchy of Phyllis's business.

The next day, I sat in a chair in front of Phyllis's desk. "I don't think it's fair that you're paying the administrative assistant more than me."

Phyllis scowled. We'd had *this* conversation before. "I suppose you ran right over and asked Stacy how much she was making!" Regardless of her annoyance, Phyllis offered to raise my salary to Stacy's, but I began again to search for another job. In late May, I saw an ad for Director of Development at The Nature Conservancy, the same job I'd interviewed for six months earlier. I called Tom, the director.

"I see the position is open again," I said. "I figured whomever you hired was incompetent, or else the job is so awful they quit."

Tom laughed. "Neither actually. We never found the right candidate."

He invited me to interview again, and so two weeks later I arranged for Steve's mother to stay with him and I drove to Lansing. This time, I was calm and composed as I shook hands with the panel of board members. After an hour of questions, Tom posed a hypothetical dilemma. "If you had to choose between visiting with a major donor who is flying into town for one day, or completing the paperwork for an annual report, what would you choose to do?"

"The donor," I replied. The answer seemed obvious.

"But the report is going to press the next day and you have hours of budget calculations. You have to get your information to the national office and you'll hold up production."

Everyone stared at me. I must have given the wrong answer. Otherwise, why was Tom raising the stakes? Still, I followed my instincts.

"You might not get another opportunity to see the donor."

The reaction of the panel was imperceptible.

"Is that the right answer?" I asked. They laughed.

"That's what I'd do," Tom said. "If you were hired," he asked, "when would you be able to start?"

"Probably not until July," I said. "I'm taking care of my boyfriend who's very ill." Cendra's line again, dusted off for this second interview.

"I apologize for being forward," Tom said, "but last November you said that you didn't expect him to live until Christmas. What happened?"

I'd completely forgotten that bit of conversation from the previous interview. How could I explain the last six months when Steve, no longer enduring chemotherapy, seemed healthier?

"He didn't die," I said.

Tom looked doubtful.

"We've contacted hospice," I said, feeling as if I were betraying Steve, speaking of him as if he were an obstacle in my career path. "He really *isn't* going to live much longer." *Don't worry sir, this time he won't be so unreliable.*

A week later I accepted the job. "You were a totally different person in this interview," Tom said after we agreed on a starting salary. I didn't explain that it was because I didn't care if I was hired or not. The job was completely unimportant, ephemeral. Jobs come and go. In the grand scheme of life and death, what's a little job?

One Saturday afternoon, Joey showed up at our door. We hadn't seen him since the night he told us about Phil's motorcycle accident. Joey's hair was cut short, his sideburns trimmed. He'd shaved his moustache and beard, and his face was white where the hair was absent, a kind of ghostly remembrance of his old self. It was the first time I'd seen his naked face, and it was like meeting him anew.

"Hey," Steve said, reaching up from the couch to shake Joey's hand. "Where have you been?"

"In a rehabilitation center," Joey said. "I work during the day, and then I go there at night and on weekends. It's over in Bridgeton."

"Is that right?" Steve said, making the effort to sit up. "That's great, Joe."

Joey described the program. He talked about his psychologist, whom he saw weekly. I'd never heard him speak so much. He was proud and excited, as if he'd discovered something new, a new person, himself.

"My counselor says I gotta get all my anger out. She says I got a lot of anger."

He inflected "anger" as if it were a tangible thing, like money, as if he were surprised to see it right in front of him, something he never knew he had. Steve had told me that Joey had been teased as a boy for his small stature, and a speech impediment. We were quiet for a few minutes, Steve and I adjusting to this new Joey, though he still tapped the ashes of his cigarette frequently, the same nervous gesture.

"There's a guy in there, an electrician named Whitey. He's drying out from alcohol. He says he knows you."

Steve thought for a minute. "I know him. He used to come to work drunk and find a hiding spot to sleep." He took a long, deliberate draw from his cigarette, as if the smoke were sustaining him. He exhaled. "I'm glad he's finally taking care of that."

"He says to say hi from the guys," Joey said. "Want me to tell him anything?"

Steve paused, and I imagined he was thinking of some other scenario that Joey could tell Whitey, who'd report back to Steve's fellow union members, something other than he'd abandoned treatment and was now waiting to die.

"Tell him hi, I guess," Steve said. "And good luck."

That was how Steve reconciled his circumstances, in terms of luck, of fate. During his final visit to Zion, he'd written in a letter to me, *I guess there are lucky people and unlucky people. I'm just one of the unlucky ones.*

In late May, we celebrated our birthdays again, though celebrate is not the right word. Steve turned thirty-one. I had no present for him. What could I give him? He needed no material objects. Instead, a month before I'd written to a consumer column in the *Ann Arbor News* to get the address of Bob Seger. My plan was to solicit seats to an upcoming sold-out concert. A woman who'd read my letter in the paper sold me her tickets, but when the concert date arrived, Steve was too ill to attend.

For my twenty-seventh birthday, Steve gave me a half-carat solitaire diamond in an 18-karat gold setting. The ring was lovely, but I broke down when I opened the box. It was an engagement ring, a vow of wedlock, an oath for the future: diamonds are forever. I was touched by Steve's gesture, especially after all we'd been through with our relationship troubles, but I was more moved because I knew how arduous it was for him to dress, to sit in an uncomfortable car, to walk around a brightly lit, crowded, labyrinthine mall. He was so weak, his skin ashen, his frame emaciated. His white smile had grayed. He'd neglected his teeth, and probably the drugs had a dulling affect. He'd lost his blonde curls with chemotherapy, and his hair, which had regrown a drab gray-brown, was oily and matted. Gary, Steve's childhood friend, who'd taken Steve shopping, told me later that in one store the salespeople had shunned them, probably mistaking Steve for an AIDS patient; in 1987, AIDS was cause for hysteria.

Steve handed me a letter with the ring, a sheet of yellow lined notebook paper folded into a tiny square, like a secret love note from a school boy. Inside, in compact tense hand-writing in red ink, he'd addressed the letter formally to Maureen, as if this were an official document:

Dear Maureen,

I pray that I could spend many more birthdays with you. It's just so hard to think that some day soon I will not be with you. I've never felt love like this before. I feel as if we are one, and when I am gone I will live through you. You are such a strong, understanding person and I have been so lucky just to know you. You have done so much for me, my kids, and family, and I am so proud of you. I know I don't tell or show you enough how much you mean to me, but I truly love you. I know this has been hard on you, so please forgive me for the bad things I've done and said. I love you so very much, Maureen, and I wish you a better, happier life.

Always remember, and never forget
I love you, Steve

When Steve accepted his fate, when he knew that separation was inevitable, he released me. He wished for me a "better, happier life." When I understood finally that I would lose Steve, I cleaved to him as he journeyed ever closer to the border between the earthly and the spirit worlds.

22. Checklist

June 1987. Sixteen months after Steve was diagnosed with cancer. He ate less, slept more, moved only from couch to recliner to bed. He didn't have the energy to work on stained glass and so left the panel he was making for me unfinished, three entwined roses framed in etched glass, his most complex project with over a hundred pieces arced and curved in degrees difficult to cut.

One day, Steve phoned everyone listed in his black address book, people he hadn't spoken to in years, women he dated before me in New York, like Theresa, the school teacher. He told everyone that he was dying, called to announce the event as if he were inviting them to his birthday party. Steve's friend, Al, with whom we'd socialized occasionally before Steve was sick, asked to speak to me after talking with Steve. "I'm really sorry I haven't been over," he said. He was seeking forgiveness for avoiding Steve during his entire illness, but I was not feeling generous. "He's not dead yet," I said. Al promised, but never visited.

By mid-month, Steve was ill enough to qualify for insurance-covered home care, though the criteria were never clearly articulated. Ingrid, the hospice director, simply deemed this. It must have been because Steve needed attendance around the clock. He was so frail, and the nausea returned, this time with blood in his vomit. His mobility declined severely. To use the bathroom, he reached his hands to me and I pulled him up from the couch. Then he stood behind me, his hands on my shoulders as if we are kids playing choo-choo train. He bore his weight on my back (at six-one, he weighed a hundred pounds, twenty pounds less than I weighed), and we lumbered slowly into the bathroom. The nursing agency set up a portable commode in the living room, but Steve preferred porcelain and plumbing. I admired his effort, in spite of the labor required, toward this small comfort, toward dignity.

Three or four nurses came and went before we found someone Steve could tolerate in the small apartment with him for hours each day. Some of the nurses talked constantly. Others watched television or knit silently, and this irked Steve, too, as if he (or they) weren't present. Finally, the agency sent a woman named Donna who had three grown sons. Donna was imperturbably jovial, though not overly so. She kept busy, but didn't ignore Steve, somehow striking the right balance.

I gave Phyllis two weeks notice, but I warned her that I might not be able to fulfill even that obligation.

"You won't just leave us hanging, will you?" she said.

"I'll try not to," I replied. It didn't matter. All I managed to accomplish at work was to sharpen pencils, organize my drawers and files, and arrange and rearrange the items on my desk, forming neat little piles.

While I was at work, Donna cooked French toast for Steve's breakfast, taking care to remove the whitish blotch from the clear albumin of the egg, and thereafter I removed this blotch too so that Steve could have perfect, blotchless French toast. Donna washed dishes and baked oatmeal cookies. She bathed Steve with warm cloths, which he hadn't allowed me to do. Somehow, in her motherly way, she overrode his protests. She was attentive, yet kept out of Steve's way, which meant that she managed, in that small apartment, to allow Steve a sense of privacy. Privacy affords dignity; to lose your privacy is to lose your self, if the self is a force in control of its bodily desires, its needs, and movement. To be constantly under surveillance, exposed, checked and monitored, looked at and touched, is to lose power, to lose freedom.

The nurses kept charts. They took Steve's pulse and blood pressure, recorded the dispensation of morphine and Dilaudid, noted his bowel movements and urine output, and wrote daily remarks on his condition, what he ate, how he felt. At night, I maintained this practice of record-keeping. It seemed important somehow, the historical noting of every fluctuation of Steve's body, as if this alone were keeping him alive.

Or perhaps this tricked my focus to the medical aspects of Steve's condition, detoured my mind from looking squarely at what was happening, that Steve was dying incrementally and I was measuring this, parsing the whole into exiguous, conceivable pieces. It gave me meaningful work, something to do. Doing nothing at all, standing by while Steve was dying made me complicit in his death: meant I allowed it. Accepted it. Maybe even desired it. Recently, I'd added a second request to my usual bed time prayer: *Please heal Steve. Or let him die.*

Donna brought me a faded checklist of signs that forecast impending death, though neither she nor any of the other nurses quantified *impending*, which could mean months, weeks, days, hours. Death would come, but when exactly? From that point on, I was on a death watch, like a tornado watch, a severe weather warning. Cyanosis was the first sign on the list, a lack of oxygen, which caused bluish extremities. Cold, clammy skin portended death, according to the checklist, as did hallucinations. A jump in pulse rate to as high as 140 was an augury. Steve's pulse varied from 90 to 120 every day, though he was phlegmatic, and rarely moved.

The death-knell which perplexed and frightened me most was Cheyne-Stokes breathing, a pattern of respiration named by two physicians in the early 1800s, which occurs most commonly in infants and in dying people: first breaths and last. Charted on a graph, Cheyne-Stokes breathing looked like a series of small sharp peaks reaching higher and higher as inhalations deepen, like stalagmites on the floor of a cave, followed by a flat line—apnea, no breathing at all. Then the pattern repeated.

I studied the graph and the written description many times, but I couldn't discern what I should *listen* for. Each night in bed I eavesdropped on Steve's breathing, which was irregular anyway, straining to distinguish a motif even more bizarre. Studying Steve's respiration terrified me, made me realize that Steve might die in bed next to me. I became petrified of waking up to a stiff, cold body. I worried that Steve would die in the middle of the night and then suddenly bolt upright like those corpses who have muscle contractions hours after death.

Fear invaded every waking moment of my life, took residence in my body. I feared ghosts and spirits, nightfall itself, the dark. Before Steve was sick, when we rented horror movies on weekends, when being frightened was pleasurable, he delighted in scaring me, lurking in the shadows while I was in the bathroom, then leaping out as I passed him, both of us laughing at how I'd jumped and screamed. I'd savor the safety of his embrace following the prank. After we watched *The Shining* one night, Steve terrified me for weeks by curling his index finger and growling, "redrum redrum redrum," like the little boy in the film.

One night, resting in bed, I said to Steve, "If you *can* come back after you die, I want you to. I want to know that you're all right. But promise you won't scare me, okay? Even if it's just a joke."

"I would never do that," he said.

Besides my fear of the occult, there was something else that frightened me, something I didn't identify until much later. I was terrified of being left alone, abandoned in the world. Coming from a family of nine, I'd rarely been alone growing up, in college or after with Steve. I hadn't experienced solitude often enough to understand why it was something I feared, but also something I needed.

Word spread that Steve was dying, actually, practically, actively dying because of course he'd been dying all along. One night, Mrs. McMahan visited. She was the mother of Gary, Steve's childhood friend who'd taken Steve shopping for my ring. She'd known Steve as a boy, a teenager, a young man. Mrs. McMahan was a lovely, kind woman, but she sat on our couch and talked until midnight, telling us about her other son's suicide years before, reliving the saga of his death, wanting, I suppose, to connect with our experience.

After she left, I sobbed, not only because of her sad story, or even ours, but because I was so tired. Often now, Steve was awake at odd hours of the night, and if he wanted to talk, I stayed up. How many more conversations would we have, after all, though lately we repeated the same ones, reminiscing about our days in New York, our weekend ski trip in the Catskills two weeks after we'd met, how he'd told the proprietor of the motel we were on our honeymoon but then had momentarily forgotten my surname when the man requested it for the register. Or the morning we'd smeared whipped cream on our bodies because it seemed sexy, but was mostly just messy. How after I left for Europe, when neither of us were sure we'd see each other again, he'd found a pair of my underwear beneath the bed and delivered them to my mother at the Hitching Post, washed and folded, in a brown paper lunch bag. He seemed so sad, my mother had told me.

Mostly we talked about the stories we used to tell each other, the paradise we'd fabricated, the country home, the garden, the bees, the honey.

"You can still do that, Mo," Steve said, one night. Under the sheet, we held hands, stared up at the ceiling.

"I don't want to do that."

"You'll find somebody else. I want you to find somebody else," he said.

"I don't want anybody else."

"I don't want you to be alone."

"I only want you," I said. "I'll never fall in love like this again."

"Yes you will."

"No I won't." It was a kind of vow, and I believed it.

My mother visited. She'd promised to come and help, and had been waiting for me to say when we needed her. "I've already spoken with my boss," she said. "I can come for the funeral if you want."

"You should see Steve before he dies," I said.

In late June, I picked my mother up at the airport in Detroit. On the drive to Saline, I prepared her for Steve's condition. "Don't talk to him too much," I warned. "He doesn't have the energy to listen. Try not to wear him out, okay?" My mother is a talker, like Mrs. McMahan, and she'd be alone with Steve during my last week of work.

Each night, my mother prepared homemade meals, my favorite foods from childhood, rich and starchy: chicken pot pie, lasagna, stuffed fried pork chops. She scrubbed our apartment until it sparkled, and even though it was a humid sticky week, she ironed all of my dresses. "Oh Mom," I said, when she proudly showed me the outfits hanging crisply in my closet. "Thank you." I didn't have the heart to tell her they'd be balled up in garbage bags when I moved after Steve died.

One morning, when my mother was taking a particularly long time in the shower, I stuck my head in the bathroom door and found her hunched on her hands and knees in the tub, scrubbing the rust ring and mildewed tiles, water raining down on her naked body. "Mom, don't bother," I pleaded. "We won't be living here much longer."

Two days after my mother arrived, I asked Steve if she was driving him crazy. "Hell no," he said. "She barely speaks to me. I say, 'Sit down and talk to me,' but she runs around cleaning all day." All of my mother's stifled talk, quashed energy, has been channeled into a cleaning blitz.

"Mom, you can *talk* to Steve," I said. "He wants you to, just don't overdo it."

In the evenings, Steve and I, huddled in bed like children, yelled to my mother in the living room. "Come talk to us. Tell us a story."

She sat at the foot of our bed and talked. *Did I tell you about Josie? Her ass is sitting in a tub of gravy. She fell off the curb in front of the Shop Rite—she was three sheets to the wind, of course, but she'll never admit* *that—and so she sued the town for failing to shovel the sidewalk and won $20,000 crying lost productivity, not that she makes it to work very often, she's always getting soused with Rose down at the Shamrock.* Aside from the customers back at The Hitching Post, my mother's patients were her favorite subject and the litany of other people's ailments in lurid medical detail recited in my mother's smooth vanilla voice, a pulsing vein of talk that lasted over an hour, lulled us, sent Steve and me drifting on a raft of words into a deep slumber. My mother's soothing hypnotic soliloquies temporarily erased from my mind the actuality of Steve's cancer, the daily bread of him dying cell by cell like a failed scientific experiment.

After my mother left, I had one month off before I started my new job at The Nature Conservancy. Donna and Ingrid from hospice and Cendra assured me that Steve would not live another month. I left the apartment only to shop for food, or to tend my tiny garden in a wooden box on the veranda. I'd planted Red Hot Sally's in honor of my sister, portulacas, a basil plant, and one broccoli. The three-by-three box was my first garden since I was ten, when my mother let me plant a row of green beans in her plot. About mid-summer that year, my beans were being decimated by insects. I found a can of Raid in the basement and read the instructions for killing garden pests: hold the can two feet from the foliage and spray lightly. In my zeal to protect my string beans, I'd saturated the leaves and overnight all my plants died. I was horrified at what I'd done.

In my puny container garden, I protected my single broccoli plant like a parent, picking off the tiny mint-green caterpillars that chewed holes in the leaves. I meticulously dead-headed my portulacas. Each flower lasted only a day, opening up to the sun, then folding up forever. The sooner I removed the browned petals, the sooner a new blossom appeared.

Aside from tending my ill-arranged garden, mostly I stayed inside as if grounded for some misbehavior. I listened to the same CD incessantly, Suzanne Vega's *Solitude Standing*, which was all over the airwaves that summer, my favorite song "Calypso," about the nymph who offered Odysseus immortality if he stayed on her island. The moody synthesizer sounded like time bending, Vega's voice a smooth rasp, *It's a lonely time ahead / I do not ask him to return / I let him go, I let him go.* That song was a too-close sound track of my life, my future.

Steve slept all but a few hours a day. He woke to smoke a cigarette, watch a show, then napped again. I couldn't read, couldn't concentrate, so most often I stared out the window as if it were a movie screen, watching the neighbor boys play army, the girls chalking wobbly squares on the sidewalk. One perfect summer day I spied two young girls across the street, watched as one girl opened her mouth wide and the other peered in, looking at a shiny silver filling, or a cavity perhaps, something or nothing. This intimacy made me wistful for childhood, before I knew anything of the world, when happiness filled that vacuum. I fantasized about being a girl, of starting all over from age eleven, before my parents divorced, before I got my period with its attendant complications of love and sex and birth and death. I felt helpless and small and alone. Not brave or courageous, as people kept saying. Only frightened.

Mid-July rolled in a heat wave. Sticky, oppressive. The air was not air but halfway to water, more than half, air that could drown you. Steve's father installed an air conditioner and we hung thick blankets in the doorways, curtaining off the bedroom and kitchen so that the living room was cool for Steve. He stayed there all morning, all day, all evening until bedtime. In the kitchen, on the other side of the blanket where Steve rarely ventured anymore, it was twenty degrees hotter, as if it were a different climate, a different longitude and latitude altogether.

We draped beach towels over the windows in the living room to block the heat and light so that Steve could sleep during the day, and with its dark paneling and brown rug, the windows opaqued, the living room became the dying room: cool, dark, static, like a theater. We watched movie after movie; sometimes I rented the same movies, which I only realized twenty minutes into the story. I forgot the titles by the next day, forgot whole plots. My mind, like an Etch-A-Sketch, shook away the fact of Steve's cancer and replaced it with the fiction of films. Then it shook that away, too.

Steve ate little, so I didn't cook. I had no appetite anyway: the heat, the rank stale smell in the apartment, the low-voltage buzzing that filled my stomach. I dropped weight quickly—five pounds, ten pounds, fifteen. I liked my smaller, lighter body, my diminished self, which had a strange spiritual quality, a lightness, like the time in college I attended a Sikh kundalini yoga retreat, took a vow of silence, ate only small quantities of rice and yogurt, rose at four in the morning to chant and stretch and pose. I felt nimble, wispish, as if I could be carried away by a strong wind. When I was very young, on gusty days I'd take my father's big black umbrella and holding it open, leap off a stone wall to see if I could float like Mary Poppins. That's how my body felt, a little hollow.

Cendra scolded me. "Think of yourself as your own child," she said. "Would you let your child eat only crackers for supper? Go three days without sleep? If you aren't healthy, how can you help Steve?" This message didn't sink into my psyche easily. Looking after myself seemed like an extra burden: two people to take care of instead of one.

23. Purple Loosestrife

Tom, my new boss, called, said it would be nice if I could attend a volunteer work day at a nature preserve near me, Ives Road Fen in Tecumseh, though I didn't officially start work for another two weeks. I didn't want to go, didn't want to subtract a day from my finite, almost calculable time left with Steve, but I agreed because Tom was my boss so he could tell me what to do. Donna, the oatmeal-cookie-baking nurse, stayed with Steve that Saturday morning. I awoke foggy-headed from my usual four hours of sleep, and running late, quickly dressed in old jeans and work boots, packed a lunch and ran out the door, forgetting to eat breakfast. The temperature outside was in the high nineties and muggy already at eight in the morning.

At the preserve, I walked down into the mushy fen—like a bog, I learned, only fed from underground springs—squashing plants, and sinking several inches into the peat, tripping over knee-high hummocks of grass. Our mission was to eradicate purple loosestrife, a blazing lilac-flowered plant that grew in profusion in wetlands. In spite of its showy beauty, purple loosestrife was a noxious invasive. A single plant released over two million seeds, which floated on water currents to colonize wetlands, choking out the delicate native species, just like the cancer cells crowded out the healthy ones in Steve's body.

Using loppers, we were to cut tall stalks of loosestrife at the base before they flowered and set seed. I surveyed the fen. The loosestrife— once I could distinguish it from similar tall fibrous stems—was everywhere. The project seemed futile, Sisyphean. The sun beat down. I hadn't thought to bring a hat or sunglasses. I sweat profusely; it must have been ninety-eight degrees. After a few hours, I began to wonder when we'd quit. I felt my stomach rumble and fold in hunger. My back ached from bending over with the awkward heavy loppers. I hadn't realized how out of shape I was, how weak. I stood to take a break and a wave of nausea rushed over me. I felt sick and lightheaded, faint. The sun glared whitely in my eyes, and then suddenly I couldn't see anything but a solid wall of dark purple-blue, like a blank television screen.

I heard someone sloshing nearby, a volunteer whose name I'd forgotten.

"Help," I said. "I don't feel good."

"Here, drink some water," she said.

"I can't see." I flailed my arms in front of me, and she placed the bottle in my hand, and I gulped and spilled water down my neck and the front of my shirt.

"I feel like I'm going to faint," I said, stooping to splash my face with cold, spring-fed water.

"Go lie down in the shade," she said.

"I can't see," I reminded her, and she took my elbow and guided me trippingly up the hill. On the way up, my hands cramped, my fingers clenching into fists. I tried to pry my fingers open, but my hands spasmed into fists again, as if I were clutching something precious, a key or a jewel. At the top of a hill, out of the fen, my vision returned. I slumped under a sprawling oak, drank more water, cooled down.

"Eat something," the volunteer said, whose name I recalled was Jenny. I forced myself to take a bite of peanut butter sandwich, which was gummy and difficult to swallow. I flexed my fingers; the cramping was gone. I felt foolish having drawn all this attention, for having collapsed from heat stress when everyone else was fine. I made excuses to the people who gathered around me. "I haven't been getting much sleep," I said. "I forgot to each breakfast."

They shook their heads. What a stupid girl, they must have thought, how careless.

Before I left, the trip leader asked if I could cart away some garbage bags filled with loosestrife. The volunteers loaded the back of Steve's pickup truck, and I drove home, my hands trembling. Donna saw that I was a wreck and immediately sent me to bed and stayed beyond her shift while I slept for hours. The bags of weeds stayed in the back of the truck for a week. When they began to smell of rot, I hauled each one, rain soaked and heavy as a corpse, to the curb for pick-up on garbage day.

The kids hadn't visited for a month since Steve's health had declined so precipitously, but one Sunday Bill and Louise dropped them off, then drove to the supermarket and the mall. Steve and Sarah stepped outside onto the veranda, further than Steve had walked in weeks. When they returned, Sarah was wiping her eyes. Embarrassed to be crying, she tried to smile and pretend that nothing was wrong. Sarah's bravery worried me. I hoped she would cry later, but I feared she never would.

Steve called Nate and Lisa over next to him where he sat in his La-Z-Boy. Sarah and I sat together on the couch. "I have something to tell you," he said.

They stood obediently near the arm of the recliner. Steve touched Nate's face, Lisa's hair. "I want you to know that I love you," he said. "But I'm not going to be around any longer."

Nate started to sniffle like when he'd been scolded.

"I want you to do good in school," Steve said to Nate, who would start first grade in a few weeks. Nate nodded and rubbed his eyes with his balled up fists.

"Lisa, you be a good girl. I love you," Steve said.

Lisa smiled her cute crooked grin. "Poor Dad," she said, and petted the top of Steve's hair with her pudgy little hand.

Steve wept just a few tears, as if he didn't have a wealth of fluid and those were his last drops and he gave them up for Sarah and Nate and Lisa.

Months later, Louise, who taught Sunday school, would explain to Lisa how Jesus died on the cross for our sins, how three days later he came back from the dead. Lisa said, "Why can't my dad come back? I want my dad to come back."

Steve didn't die on schedule and I had to start my new job. For a week, I drove eighty miles from Saline to Lansing, worked eight hours, then drove home, exhausted and headachy from all the reading and learning and thinking. Nobody mentioned Steve at my new job, not April or Dave or Betty, my coworkers, or Tom, my boss, because they didn't know him, and the not-knowing erased him. I was in my future already, my new Steve-less life, until I drove home to the past where Steve was still living, still dying.

Steve wrote another poem, this time abandoning rhyme and narrative for simile. What escape was left a dying man but the disguise of metaphor?

Burning down, down, down, down
as the candle burns smaller
the flame begins to flicker
until it burns out.

You can light another candle
it will do the same
my life is like a candle
it has started to flicker.

I envisioned Steve sitting on the couch, smoking a cigarette, staring at a candle, watching the wax drip, the stem shrink, the dance of the flame wild and erratic as it guttered. When I was a child and my family attended Mass, I believed that the votive candles near the altar in church—prayers for those who were suffering—had to be kept lit for the benediction to work, and I worried about what would happen if the candles blew out. It seemed such a precarious ritual, that a flame vulnerable to any stirring of the air was all that carried hope forward.

24. In the Dawn He Sails Away

In the dawn he sails away / to be gone forever more
Suzanne Vega, "Calypso"

Friday evening I returned home from work to find Louise, who'd stayed with Steve that day, in the kitchen packing dishes in cardboard boxes, glassware, and the jars of tomatoes that Steve and I had canned two years before. Who'd have thought they'd last so long?

"I want to go home," Steve had said that morning, and so after packing all night, we moved to Steve's parents' house, his childhood home, the house into which he was born, where he grew into a young man, the house he left behind at eighteen when he ventured forth into his own life. Steve's parents forfeited their bedroom for Steve and me, and moved into Louise's sewing room for the time being. My commute to Lansing was halved, so I could sleep a bit later in the mornings, arriving home in time for the dinners Louise fixed.

All week I sensed that Steve was going to die on the weekend. I knew that he wanted me with him when he left, not at work, or idling at a red light, picking up bread or milk, or standing in line at the bank. On Saturday, the first of August, Steve's pulse jumped from 120, where it had been for six weeks, to 140, nearly twice the normal pulse rate in an adult male, 72 beats per minute, slightly slower in tall people like Steve, slower yet when one is sitting as opposed to standing, slowest when a body is recumbent, as Steve was nearly every hour of every day. Inside Steve's body, while he slept, his heart revved, pumping as if he were sprinting.

His skin was clammy, another sign on the checklist, like all the clichés. He'd been cool and moist for a couple of days, like a basement wall on a humid summer day. Steve's father installed an air conditioner for Steve, but despite the gelid temperature and his cool skin, Steve was thirsty, desperately thirsty. All afternoon on Saturday, Louise crushed ice for Steve's juice, though she could never meet his discriminating specifications. He'd take a sip from the tumbler, then hand it back to his mother. "Too big," he'd say, sending her back into the kitchen to pound ice.

"Pulverize it!" he yelled from the bedroom, and we smiled conspiratorially. It seemed funny, his mother in the kitchen pulverizing ice, the birr of the blender in the background. Still, we couldn't slake Steve's thirst, and so after dinner I drove to the convenience store on the corner and bought a large blueberry slush, which was perfect, except it turned his lips and tongue blue, the color of his toes, which was another sign on the checklist: cyanosis.

At eleven o'clock Steve's parents retreated into their room, his mother without her glasses, bags under her eyes, blinking, in her daintily-flowered nightgown down to her toes; his father still in his work clothes, an old pair of jeans that sagged. We said goodnight and I closed the bedroom door. I helped Steve up from the recliner into bed, and fixed five pillows around him, as had become our nightly ritual: one under his head, a second between his skinny legs to keep his knees from jabbing, a third he hugged to his chest, and two more wedged behind his back to prop him on his side, the position which afforded sleep.

I climbed in beside Steve, kissed his cheek, said "I love you." Turned off the light.

A minute later, Steve asked, "What's burning?"

"Nothing," I said, sniffing the air.

"Who's frying something?"

"Nobody," I said.

"I smell something frying."

"I don't know what it is, Steve." I squeezed his hand.

"What's frying?" he asked again.

I remembered that hallucinations were on the checklist, though I hadn't imagined olfactory ones.

Steve was restless. He wanted to go back to the recliner, so I turned on the light and helped him walk the few steps to the La-Z-Boy and arranged his pillows and afghan. A few minutes later, I heard him rustling in his chair, trying to get up. He wanted to get back into bed, and so he leaned on me and we trudged to the bed. I rolled over to sleep, but almost immediately Steve wanted to sit in the recliner again. I helped him stand, but halfway to the chair his knees buckled and he collapsed. "Steve!" I yelled, half-carrying, half-dragging his withered body to the recliner.

His parents heard me and ran into the room, wrapping their robes around themselves.

"I think he's dying," I said.

Steve called out. "Mom. Dad."

"We're here, honey," his mother said.

He closed his eyes.

I was momentarily jealous. Why hadn't he called my name? Then I felt awful and guilty for my pettiness. Of course he would call for his parents as he lay dying, those who brought him into the world, whose bodies created him. Still, I rationalized, he didn't call my name because he *knew* I was there next to him, as I had been nearly every night for the last eighteen months of his illness, and two years before as his lover.

I bent to Steve's ear and whispered, "In case I don't see you again, I love you," similar to what I'd said when I left for Europe, leaving open the possibility of reunion. I felt like I was arming him with ruby slippers, that wherever he was going, he'd take my love with him, as if love was a force. I kissed Steve on the cheek, and he squeezed my finger, and he seemed fine for little while. It was midnight, and I called the local hospice, which was staffed entirely by volunteers, unlike the paid nurses at Ingrid's agency in Ann Arbor. We'd alerted them when we arrived at Steve's parent's house, but we hadn't needed their help in the week we'd been in town, so none of the volunteers knew us.

A woman answered the phone, and I told her my name, and Steve's. "I think he's dying," I said. "What should we do?"

"What's going on?" she asked. I told her his pulse rate, how he was cold and clammy. I asked her if this meant that he was close to death.

"It could be days," she said.

"Well…" I didn't know what else to say.

"What do you want me to do?" she asked.

"I guess we just wanted some reassurance."

"There's really nothing I can do," she said. "You don't really want me to come out there, do you?"

"I don't know." I didn't know anything at that moment. I felt completely unsure of what was happening in spite of the obvious signs. All the reading I'd done, the care I'd given Steve, nothing prepared me for his actual death. "Just keep doing what you're doing," the hospice woman said. "Give me a call back later if anything changes." I hung up and walked back into the bedroom.

Steve complained that his stomach hurt, and began to whimper, then moan softly. He hadn't eaten much in the previous two weeks, nor had a bowel movement in as long. I gave him an extra shot of morphine by pressing the button on his IV unit, but his stomach cramps intensified. He clutched his abdomen and groaned. "Mo," he said quietly, "I think I shit my pants."

I saw black fluid in his underwear, the blue and red and yellow polka-dot boxer shorts from his cousin Jessica. He'd worn them for the last two weeks. They were loose and comfortable, and there seemed to be no point in changing each day, effortful as that was. I took off his shorts and cleaned him up. He continued moaning loudly, then louder still. He moaned and moaned until his breathing became moaning and each exhale was a loud wail, a long, sonorous ululation, like the slow stroke of horse hair across the strings of a cello.

I rubbed his abdomen vigorously to stimulate movement in his bowels. A friend in college had taught me colonic massage, how to knead clockwise, following the layout of the large intestine.

"Are you sure that's not hurting him?" Louise said.

"I don't think so." I continued to massage Steve, and black fluid trickled out of him.

"Can you get me some warm washcloths," I said to Louise and Bill, who were standing near Steve's chair.

I placed a large disposable pad under him. More black liquid the color of old car oil poured out of him. The odor wasn't foul, but it smelled like guts, a cow liver, or internal organs. As rapidly as the fluid gushed out of Steve's body, I tried to wipe him clean, but it was gushing too quickly. I asked his father to get me a cup to catch the liquid, and a bucket to dump it in. His mother rinsed washcloths and kept me supplied with clean, warm towels. Steve's eyes rolled back into their sockets, and he moaned loudly and steadily, rhythmically.

His father returned from the kitchen with a Styrofoam cup, which I placed under Steve. The cup snapped in half.

"For God's sake, Bill, get something that won't break," Louise said.

He returned with a small flowered teacup. Louise looked at him in exasperation, but I took the teacup. It worked.

The black liquid abated somewhat and I cleaned Steve, wiped his sweaty face and wrapped him in another diaper. But then the flow began again. Each time the liquid stopped, I thought surely that was the end of it, but the black fluid kept coming, like the sins of his life, thirty-one years of sins pouring out of his body.

Steve was bellowing now, loudly and steadily. I couldn't stand that he was in so much pain, so I pushed the button for another bolus of morphine, but that didn't help. He moaned and bayed like a sickly animal. I prepared a syringe of valium, though he wasn't due for a shot.

"I don't think you better give him more so soon," Louise said.

I poked the needle into the rubber stopper on the tiny vial of Valium, while Louise read the fine print that accompanied each bottle.

"It says here that he could overdose."

"I don't think it will make a difference." I tapped the bubbles and inserted the needle into the port in Steve's leg.

"An overdose could lead to a heart attack," Louise read.

"That would be a blessing," I said, and pushed the plunger, watched the fluid drain into the syringe in Steve's thigh. Immediately he began to hyperventilate, his rapid breaths accompanied by a dry rasping sound as if he were straining for air. *Oh my God*, I thought. *His mother is right. I've killed him.* But the fit passed after a minute and Steve's moaning resumed, low steady bursts of noise that sounded now like a foghorn whose generator was running down.

For the moment, Steve was clean and dry.

Bill brewed coffee and poured it into a beat-up green metal thermos that he carried around with him. I'd always wondered if he added whiskey or something stronger to the coffee, but nobody in Steve's family ever mentioned the ubiquitous thermos. Louise filled syringes with Valium, neatly arranging a supply for the next four days.

"I don't think you need to bother," I said, but she was intent, and I felt a pang of tenderness for her.

Steve was pressing his hand on his abdomen, whimpering. He must be impacted, I thought, the blockage the source of his pain. It had happened before. I put on surgical gloves and inserted a finger in his rectum. I could feel the obstruction, and began to pull out masses of sludge, which undammed the passage and freed more black liquid. I pulled out more hard balls, massaging Steve's abdomen with my other hand. Black liquid effused from his body.

"I don't know how you can do that," Louise said. She sat by Steve's side and wiped his brow. On this, Steve's last day of his life, I felt able to do anything for him, to suffer with him, the meaning of compassion, to love him body and soul, to help him die, whatever that might take. I wanted him to know, before he left this world, what love was.

After a while the blockage seemed cleared and the flow of black liquid ceased. Steve's moaning softened into tremulous breathing, which gave way finally to a gentle, steady respiration. I wiped his face, cleaned him up, and hoped that we could sleep a bit. Louise picked up towels and dropped them in the laundry hamper. Bill lit a cigar, coughed up phlegm, spit into his handkerchief.

I closed the door to our bedroom. Steve was in his La-Z-Boy, clean, diapered, afghan across his lap, resting his head on his favorite feather pillow. The clock on the wall just above his chair read 5:02 a.m., which surprised me, that so much time had passed. I scanned the room, the half-full glasses on the night table, plastic wrappers on the aquamarine shag carpet, Chux pads and rubber gloves and syringes. The mess could wait until the morning.

I sighed and looked at Steve. His eyes were shut, and he seemed to be sleeping peacefully. Then I noticed a strangeness, an absence of movement. His bony chest was not rising or falling. His eyes were not skittering beneath his lids. He was perfectly still. *He's dead,* I thought. I felt stunned in spite of the five hours that had just passed. I felt for his pulse, first at his wrist, and then by pushing my thumb hard against his jugular.

Still.

I called his mother and father. "Come in here," I said. "I think he's dead."

I pressed my ear to Steve's chest. There was no sound, not even faintly, not even an echo.

"Get a mirror," I said. His mother brought one, and I held it under Steve's nose, but no mist appeared. I fell to my knees.

Steve's father said, "Son of a bitch," then punched the wall. His knuckles began to bleed, and he wept. His mother cried into a towel, and then we all three hugged.

Louise called the funeral home. As I waited for the undertaker, I stood staring out the picture window in the living room, at the mist swarming the lawn. Phyllis, my former boss, who'd studied classics, had told me of a myth in which mist was the sky separating from his lover, water, after a night of mingling in love. The grass was silvered with dew, tears of Aurora, the Roman goddess of dawn who wept each sunrise for her dead son, Memnon. More deaths occurred in that transition between night and morning, I'd read somewhere, as if the shift from dark to light was a changing of guards, an opportunity for souls to slip away unnoticed.

All along I'd thought that when Steve died, I'd see a filmy wraith float away from him heavenward, his spirit ascending: pneuma, the soul. The Greeks believed it departed the dying person as a sough from the mouth. I'd envisioned such a moment, crystalized, dramatized with clearly recognizable Cheyne-Stokes suspiration, Steve's chest heaving as his heart pounded its final beats, like in the movies perhaps. I thought I would know.

Instead Steve died for five hours, five long hours of suffering, his body failing. For five hours Steve died, but really only one second because he was alive, his heart beating, blood pulsing through his veins, breath on his lips until that one second, that second I looked away, when I sat on the edge of the bed and glanced around the room, rested.

He left without me after all.

PART III

25. Monochrome

Louise and I shopped for a casket in the showroom of the funeral home, like looking at furniture, a couch, something in which to rest. We selected a beautiful silk-lined cherrywood box, gleaming with polish, elegant enough to furnish your living room. Steve had talked about cremation to save money mainly, but his mother wouldn't consider it as that wasn't Christian. Of course, we couldn't buy the least expensive coffin. We'd seem cheap, as if Steve would know that we'd skimped and feel slighted.

Afterward, sitting in leather chairs in the funeral home director's office, we chose music for the service, psalms to read, and the director drafted the obituary for the newspaper. He asked whom Steve was survived by, and Louise named Sarah and Nate and Lisa, she and Bill, Karen and Linda. Each had a term to describe their relationship to Steve: daughter, son, mother, father, sister.

"And what should we call you?" the director asked.

Girlfriend seemed too juvenile.

"Special friend?" the director suggested.

"Fiancé," Louise said, and it was resolved. Steve and I were officially engaged, at least for the newspaper, posthumously, not in the nuptials section but the obits.

At home, Louise asked me to select clothes for Steve to wear. I wanted to dress him in his favorite ecru cotton sweater, a gift I'd given him one Christmas. He'd looked so handsome in that sweater, but it was August and swelteringly hot, so I put him in a short sleeve cotton dress shirt that buttoned down the front. It didn't occur to me for days that he could have worn the sweater, that temperature didn't matter. The shirt I buried Steve in was creped, a style popular for the moment, but when it faded from fashion a season later, I regretted that I hadn't dressed him in something more stylishly enduring.

The funeral was held at the Lutheran Church in his hometown. My father flew out, and he and Sally drove up from Ann Arbor, and we sat with Bill and Louise in the front row. The kids were in the balcony with their mother, far up and away. I was surprised to see the church packed with people. I didn't know who they were, or who'd told them Steve had died, how everyone had found out so soon, just one day later.

The minister didn't know Steve, but someone had given him some notes, which he incorporated into his eulogy, and I felt ashamed that I hadn't written something personal and lovely for Steve, given all the time I'd had, knowing this day would come. In the row behind me, Steve's Aunt Ethel sat with her family, and when the organist played the hymns, her voice rose above everyone else's, a piercing column of soprano, and I imagined Steve's spirit lifted by her powerful voice straight up to heaven.

After the service, I walked down the aisle, held upright by my father's strong arm around my shoulder, clutching Sally's hand, past rows of electricians, people I recognized from picking Steve up at work or union picnics we'd gone to, and I wondered who'd called them. In the parking lot, I saw Joey. The day was bright and sunny, ninety degrees, but he was wearing a long-sleeved black shirt buttoned up to his neck, black tie, black pants, black shoes. I'd worn a peach skirt and a sleeveless blouse; I'd heard that it wasn't necessary to wear black anymore, and I thought that a pastel would symbolize my gratitude that Steve's pain had ended.

But I was glad that Joey had covered himself in the monochrome of grief, black: the absence of a single color, the presence of all colors, empty and full at once. I appreciated that Joey suffered the heat in honor of Steve. Joey looked heart-broken, though underneath his sadness he seemed healthy and well, his hair neatly trimmed. We hugged each other tightly. I'd never touched him before, and I could feel his rib cage, his chest rising and falling.

I saw Deborah, Steve's ex-wife, the mother of his children. I'd never met her, or seen her up close. We hugged, and I noticed for the first time her lovely green eyes. In the basement of the church, volunteers and family friends served a potluck. Someone brought a sheet cake and there were noodle salads. Children ran around the tables and chairs. Some people ate, though I wondered how anyone could have an appetite. I couldn't imagine being hungry ever again.

People I didn't know approached me to say they were sorry, and Steve's mother and Aunt Ethel introduced me to second cousins and distant uncles, and neighbors and family friends, a whole world of people grieving Steve that I hadn't known existed.

"This is Steve's fiancé," Louise would say. "She's an absolute saint."

"God sent her to Steve," Aunt Ethel would add.

When I heard them say this, I thought of the night Steve called for me from the living room where he was resting on the couch, and I pretended not to hear him, so tired I was, in bed already and nearly asleep. And another night when I was desperate for rest, and needed to be able to function at work the next day, I said to Steve lying next to me chanting his pain, "Could you be a little more quiet?" I thought of our fights, my petty comments about his will. I felt like a fraud as I shook the hands of grieving relatives, received their sympathy, allowed Steve's mother and aunt to beatify me.

On Monday morning, I called my boss, Tom, who said, "Why don't you take the week off?" I was grateful that I did not have to ask. I flew back to Boston with my father and spent the week immersed in the care and compassion of my family in my childhood home, the home I'd left behind four years earlier, full of hope and ambition and excitement and love, to start my life with Steve.

26. California

One night in seventh grade I went skating with my friends on Memorial Pond, a tiny puddle across from Blessed Sacrament church. The night was clear and cold, and after a couple of hours my feet froze solid in my white figure skates. I had stayed out long past the point of practicality waiting for a boy named Paul to glide with me to a small island and kiss me (he did, finally). When I took my skates off, my toes were numb. At home, my mother rubbed my feet in her warm hands and when my toes began to thaw, the ache set in.

That's what it felt like after Steve died. After taking care of business matters—selecting a casket, making small talk at the service, choosing a headstone—and after the hot August days turned cool in September, I awoke to the realization of the foreverness of Steve's absence. What nobody told me when Steve was ill—not Cendra, not the hospice nurses, not my mother or father, not Pastor Scanlon—what none of them said was that when Steve's pain ended, mine would begin. I did not know about grief. Until Steve's, I'd been to one funeral in my life, for my great Uncle Patrick, which I attended when I was twelve. At the Irish wake, all my relatives were talking and drinking like it was a party, and this conviviality provided me with an opportunity to kneel at the casket as if in prayer and emotionlessly study the small stitches in my great uncle's lips. I felt no sorrow at the death of an old man who'd been a stranger to me.

Grief surprised me. Death is so commonplace; so many people die in so many various ways every minute, every second, all over the world, 150,000 people daily, an entire city of souls. Yet until it is experienced, grief is almost wholly unimaginable. Once loss is personal, grief transubstantiates into compassion. "Water is taught by thirst," Emily Dickinson wrote. Compassion is taught by grief, I learned. Our hearts are made tender by pain.

I'd imagined that after Steve died, I'd feel the opposite of grief. I thought I'd be relieved that his suffering was over, that I could get on with my life. I thought that witnessing Steve suffer and die was as sorrowful as sorrow could be. I did not imagine that I would wish Steve were still alive, wish I was still taking care of him, wish my life was once again filled with just that. As awful as it was at times, it seemed better than being left behind, empty and alone. I ached for Steve.

I had no inkling of the profundity of grief, nor the power of denial.

For months, I could not accept that Steve was gone *forever*, that he would *never* come back. Often, I caught myself thinking that he was just in California, like one of those husbands who goes to the corner store for milk or cigarettes and never returns. If I saw a lanky blue-jeaned form of a man with blonde curls pushing a cart in front of me in the supermarket, my heart clenched. I'd be surprised a second later when a stranger turned around. *Where's Steve?* I wanted to ask the imposter.

I wrote letters to Steve every night for months, a way of keeping him in my life, as poet Linda Pastan wrote: "When I describe your absence / here you are with me on the white sheets of paper." Over and over I'd write, *where are you?* And then I'd have to remind myself: *Steve is dead. He's dead. Dead.* I wrote it dozens of times in my journal, like in seventh grade when I printed the name of the boy I admired a thousand times on blue-lined paper, each repetition like a single tap in a beat I strained to hear. But even as I repeated those words like a refrain, writing in my journal with the soft lead of pencil, I couldn't help but deny the truth, keep Steve alive. Steve is dead. *Is*: the present tense of *to be*. Denial is embedded in the architecture of our language.

Tibetan Buddhists believe that a person who dies travels a perilous path between death and rebirth into another womb, a forty-nine day journey with three stages: the moment of dying; the interstice between death and the next life, called the bardo; and rebirth. If the deceased is unskilled in meditation and thus does not know where he is during the bardo, there are clues. When he walks in the sand or snow, he leaves no footprints. Under the sun, he casts no shadow. He is a ghost.

Shortly after Steve died, I had a vivid dream. In the dream, Steve was healthy, bearded as he was in winters, smiling impishly, pretending to be asleep. My blue patchwork quilt was tucked under his chin, exactly as it was in a photo I'd shot while he napped one day in my room in New York when we first met, except in my dream, Steve was lying in a mahogany casket in a room with velvet curtains and plush dark carpet. I stood on a balcony four feet above, looking down upon him in the center of the room. The balcony ran along all four walls of the room, but there were no stairs, so I could not get to Steve. Still, he knew I was there. I said, "I love you, Steve."

He said, "I love you too, Mo."

I said, "Goodbye, Steve."

He said, "Goodbye, Mo." Then he closed his eyes, and pressed his cheek to the pillow as if to sleep, and I turned and walked out of the room.

When I woke up, I knew that Steve had visited me, a necessary stop on his path to rebirth, closure. He appeared in a dream so as not to frighten me, as he'd promised, but the dream was so vivid and sharp and real that all day and into the next day I had a physical, bodily sensation of his presence.

27. Driving and Crying

I moved into my room at Sally's house in Ann Arbor, the one I'd been paying for all along. I was thankful that this room was waiting for me, that I had a place to go, to live. Each morning, I drove an hour to my new job in Lansing and focused on work for eight hours, repressing thoughts of Steve. At five o'clock, I'd barely turn out of the parking lot before I began sobbing. I wept for sixty miles, oblivious to the external world: my car a capsule, my anguish contained by its steel shell. Often when my reverie broke I failed to recognize where I was, and had to wait for a billboard or exit sign to place myself. Sometimes I discovered that I'd been driving eighty miles an hour, or forty-five. Often, I wondered how I arrived home alive. The floor of my car was littered with balled up tissues. "Gross," Sally said when she sat in the passenger seat one day. She must have thought I had a preternaturally long cold.

It seemed fitting to grieve in my car. If I were in Colorado, I'd go to the mountains. In Massachusetts, to the ocean. In Michigan, that flat land of pavement and six-lane highways and monolithic General Motors and Ford factories and a five-story-tall tire replica along the freeway toward the Motor City, my grieving seemed regionally appropriate. The daily hour of mourning for Steve in my car was our private time, he in spirit, in memory, I in body: alone and together.

I was not the only one driving and crying. There were others whose lovers or spouses had died, who cruised the highways weeping, I learned when I joined a bereavement group that Cendra recommended, a group for young widows and widowers, that is, those under the age of forty-five. I was allowed to join even though I was not technically a widow. I had the diamond from Steve as shibboleth, but even without the ring I'm sure the group would have allowed me to participate. They were a very supportive support group. Every Tuesday evening, a dozen or so young widows and widowers sat on tastefully upholstered furniture in the living room of a woman whose husband had died three years earlier. She turned her loss into a career as a grief counselor: in death she'd found her calling. Sipping coffee and tea and sniffling quietly, we took turns narrating our sad stories.

When a freshly-widowed person joined the group for the first time, the regulars turned over the floor. Often, listening to these newly wrought tales occupied the entire evening, and for that short while the rest of us could forget our own stories. Every week I thought that each new loss sounded worse than mine, and that I should be thankful that I was not, for example, the middle-aged woman whose husband and daughter had both died of cancer. Listening to that woman speak, my own loss seemed Lilliputian, a relief for which I felt guilty: she paid a high price for my perspective.

At twenty-seven, I was not the youngest in the group. There was a handsome, square-jawed college senior with a standard barber-shop trim that, together with his black-framed glasses, epitomized "clean-cut." The clean-cut man (I want to write *boy*) attended only once. He sat in an armchair and speaking softly and without inflection as if in a trance, re-enacted his fiancé's drowning. "She wasn't a very strong swimmer," he said. "Lake Michigan can fool you."

He was right. Weather conditions on the Great Lakes can shift quickly. I remember swimming in Lake Michigan once on vacation with Steve. At dusk, the surface of the lake was so placid it looked like flat earth. I cut one long, slow lap parallel to the shore, staring at blurry rocks on the sandy bottom, my goggles fogged. By the time I popped my head out of the water, a mist had stealthily surrounded me. Over my head and directionless, I couldn't tell through the mist which way was the beach, which way was Wisconsin a hundred miles across the lake. I called to Steve, and his voice like a siren lured me ashore.

"It was a sudden squall," the young man in the group said. "The waves were over six feet high. I saw her struggling and swam in after her." He pulled his fiancé onto the sand and gave her mouth-to-mouth resuscitation. "Her face was as blue as my jeans," he said. But his efforts failed and this he would know for the rest of his life. Who could write a story so cruel, I thought, so poignant as that of a young man with his drowned lover in his arms, trying to kiss her back to life, to give her breath of his own?

Gwen, a tall, slope-shouldered woman in her mid-thirties, lost her airline pilot husband. "I always kissed him goodbye," she told me, "in case the plane went down." One morning as her husband drove to work, a branch fell onto his car the exact second he passed underneath and crushed his skull. I listened to Gwen's story many times, every excruciating detail as she and I spent time together outside of the group in extracurricular mourning, commiserating over ice cream at Bob's Big Boy, feeding off each other's sadness. We had more to be miserable about, we concurred, since we did not have children, the ultimate souvenirs of a relationship.

There were two camps within the group: those whose spouses had died quickly (the aneurysms, heart attacks, car accidents, and bizarre mishaps), and those whose loved one suffered and lingered (cancer exclusively in this group). I thought I was being gracious when I said to the others, "Be thankful you didn't have to watch him suffer." And those widows and widowers replied, "Yes, that must have been difficult, but at least you had a chance to say your good-byes."

Envy exists even in grief. One can envy a death.

I participated in the support group for about eight months, until I just didn't have the energy to partake of reliving death on a weekly

basis anymore. I stopped calling Gwen. I couldn't bear how we reeked
of sadness, and outside of misery, we had little in common.

On Fridays, I saw Cendra. "Will this pain ever go away?" I asked.

"Eventually and never," she said. "It's like looking at a painting.
Every time you see it, it will be just as intense. But as time goes on, you'll
look at it less and less."

A long time passed before I understood her analogy. Looking at a
painting is a voluntary act. Grief taps what Jung called the chthonic part
of our mind, that which is linked to nature. Death, like birth, reduces
us to our biological selves, evokes primal instincts, a return to a place
and time before the names of things. In the months following Steve's
death, grief ambushed me, sucker-punched me, like the day at work
when I came upon the zip code and the name of our town, Saline, on a
bulk mailing I was preparing. It stopped me cold that Saline, Michigan
48176 continued to exist, that people still lived there, received mail, as
if nothing had changed.

Another day when I was commuting to work on I-96, a four
lane highway, the car ahead of me hit a woodchuck waddling across
the lane and squashed its hind legs. The creature frantically dragged
itself towards the shoulder of the road as my car passed over it with a
sickening thunk. I sobbed for half an hour. I felt like that creature, adrift
in a sea of fast moving objects. Stricken.

Sometimes at night, grief blew in like a quick summer storm and
only my mother could console me then. I'd dial her number, but when
she said "hello" I couldn't speak. I was sucking in a huge gulp of air,
choking on oxygen. My mother knew it was me. *It's alright now, it's okay,*
she'd say, and then great sobs let loose from my body like chunks of ice
calving off an iceberg: not words or intelligible sounds but something
primordial, unrecognizable noises from the umbilical center of my gut,
the diaphragm, the solar plexus, like someone had kicked me hard in

the stomach. The sound of air expanding the cavity in my chest and then being forced out past the catgut of my vocal chords—that was the sound my mother heard. It was a frightening sound, ugly, but the grief was pure and clean.

Through the thickness of it, the viscosity, my mother would segue from soothing words into stories, the chronicles of her life and those around her.

You know the girl who works in medical records, the cute little brunette, Suzanne? Well she got herself pregnant. The doctors told her if her multiple sclerosis got worse she couldn't have kids, so she decided it's now or never, but suddenly her boyfriend doesn't want anything to do with the kid. I don't know what she sees in that dodo.

I listened to my mother's lovely voice, not high-pitched or breathy, not low and raspy, but a smooth, clear singing speech almost, like rap but without the edges and less iambic. She rarely stammered or stuttered, uttered ers or ahs or ums. She barely paused, but she inflected and repeated and talked fast—allegro, jolly in Italian—music to my ears. In minutes, I'd be lying on my bed with the phone pressed to my ear, becalmed. My mother's words, like empty boats, floated my sadness away.

28. Jitterbug

Eight months after Steve died, I bought a bungalow on Denver Street in a so-so neighborhood in Lansing; for down payment, I used $4000 that Steve had bequeathed me. When I first moved in, I felt like I was staying in a luxury hotel, a suite of rooms. The plush wall-to-wall carpet hushed everything and made me feel like an adult and a consumer and an American. Inside I still felt like a girl, scared and uninitiated. There were things I did not know about, things I did not know how to do. I spent a month agonizing over lawn mowers. Twice or three times a week I shopped for a mower, inspecting dozens of models (for what qualities, I was never sure): cheap ones, electric ones, self-propelled; mowers with bags on the side, bags on the back, and ones with big back tires like old-fashioned baby carriages. I couldn't decide. Mechanical objects had been Steve's domain.

For two weeks, Tom, my new boss, drove to my house on Saturday to cut my lawn. One day I realized that I could not take advantage of his kindness even one more time, so I drove to Bill's Tractor Sales down the street and bought a shiny candy-apple red Snapper with a bag in the back for collecting clippings. It cost $400 and was the first item I ever purchased with a credit card. I'd selected the expensive Snapper because the guy at the store who had a burning cigarette stuck to his lip—a guy who could smoke a whole cigarette with no hands—said it would start up on the first pull every time. I'd pictured myself yanking a starter cord again and again in my front yard, as I remember my father doing, with the neighbors watching, the two bachelors across the street, childhood friends who'd moved in together after their divorces. They sat on their porch every night in easy chairs with batting busting from the seams, drinking beer, the lit end of their cigarettes like fireflies in the dark.

This made me feel like crying. For months after Steve died, any time I couldn't do something mechanical, or lift something heavy, or repair something, I cried. I helped Steve fight for his life, but I couldn't lift a cement slab in my back yard or fix a leak in my roof. One day I bought a picnic table and had it loaded into my car at the store. When I got home, I realized that I couldn't lift the box out of my car. It finally occurred to me to open the box and carry each piece separately to my backyard. I spent hours figuring out how to put the picnic table together, and proudly assembled all the legs for the table and four benches. But when I tried to attach the legs to the table top, I discovered that I'd screwed all of them together backwards. I ran inside my house and threw myself on my bed and sobbed. Later, I walked back outside and unscrewed the benches and started over.

Once I was grounded in my new house in Lansing, once I no longer spent two hours each day in the interstitial space of my car, the fog of grief began to lift and I saw myself again. I'd spent so much time looking at Steve, attending to his physical needs that I'd forgotten my own. One day I looked closely at my teeth and saw grayish purple shadows near the gum line, stains from tea, from never flossing, from foregoing the dentist for two years. I discovered new cross-hatching near my eyes, like the delicate crazing on antique pottery, and around my mouth were two creases that channeled salty tears.

As if in defiance against the assault on Steve's body, I fortified mine. Four times a week I swam at the YMCA. I'd begin my first length of crawl slowly, gliding past elderly ladies treading the shallow end in their old-fashioned bathing suits and rubber caps. After one or two laps, my breathing found a rhythm, my muscles stretched and relaxed, my lungs adjusted to this new element, this heavier air. Then I'd unspool the filmstrip in my head. I'd start with the day Steve walked into the Hitching Post, then review scenes in chronological order instead of leap-frogging to my favorite moments, recalling our New York days when we'd fallen in love, never scenes of Steve with cancer. As I steadied the pace of my laps the film in my mind flickered along. A flip-turn at the end of the pool to rewind the reel, and I'd begin again. I'd swim forty laps, always thinking of Steve, savoring our kisses over and over like a junkie, obsessing, holding him prisoner in my mind, memorizing him.

But after several months, this changed. The images began to slip from my mind. I couldn't hold on to them, as if I were swimming in the River Lethe, the mythological river in Hades whose water caused forgetfulness. When I tried to force my thoughts back to our New York days, my body—my lungs, my muscles—pulled my attention away. The water rinsed my mind clear. I felt and heard only my own heart pounding, the expansion of my lungs. Swimming was perfect solitude. Underwater, I could not cry.

I learned years after Steve died that I did all of the things one is *not* supposed to do while grieving. In bereavement, one should stay still, avoid major decisions or changes, find solace in home, routine, familiarity. Instead, I moved to a city where I knew no one, bought a house in a random neighborhood, started a new job working with strangers who scarcely knew my history. One day at work, a lovely arrangement of flowers was delivered for me. My coworkers chided me. They thought I had a lover, or a secret admirer. For a fleeting second, I too hoped that they were from some reticent suitor, but I knew before I looked at the card that the bouquet was from Steve's parents memorializing the first anniversary of his death.

Steve's mother called and wrote to me frequently, but I didn't see Steve's family often. Deborah, Steve's ex-wife, forbade me to have contact with the kids, which multiplied my grief. For a while, I saw Sarah and Nate and Lisa only in my dreams, but over time even those visitations ended. My friend, Greta, my coworker from Phyllis's company, invited me for dinner on a Friday night once, after I'd driven to Ann Arbor for counseling with Cendra. After that, twice a month I'd see Cendra, then dine with Greta and her husband, a generosity I never returned, though I believe Greta understood why I was not capable of reciprocating.

I spent many weekends with Sally, until she moved back east with her new love, her future husband, a year after Steve's death. Michigan felt strange without Steve, without Sally. In spite of its eleven million people, Michigan was for me a state filled with absence. I still had the t-shirt Steve had given me before I left for Europe, the one that read: *someone misses me in Michigan,* which I'd worn faithfully when we were continents apart. After Steve died, I never wore that shirt again. Now I was the one left behind in Michigan with nothing but a t-shirt inscribed with longing.

Alone in Lansing, I tried to construct a new, solo life, to assemble component parts—neighbors, friends, community, though I felt unschooled in this endeavor. I signed up for evening classes, Creative Writing, and Taoism, color-coding blocks in my calendar, leaving no space empty for grief to billow in like smoke and suffocate me. I felt fumbly and self-conscious, as if permanently embarrassed or scarred in some way. I thought that people could tell just by looking at me that I was marked, damaged, jinxed.

I felt unwhole. I kept trying to repair something that I thought was broken, to reassemble something that never was. I didn't understand why my expectations—what was *supposed* to happen to me, what seemed to happen to everyone else—were never realized. At the YMCA I thought I would meet friends, kindred spirits, but I liked to swim when the pool was uncrowded, when the patrons were mostly retired people, red-faced, pot-bellied old men who eyed me in my Speedo that clung like a second skin.

I imagined that after I moved into my house, neighbors would appear on my doorstep bearing casseroles and baked goods. I awaited a call from the Welcome Wagon, which as a kid I'd pictured as a Conestoga wagon driven by bonneted frontier women. I expected these things to happen on their own, as if someone else was scripting the drama of my life.

But instead, most of my neighbors remained strangers. I didn't know their surnames, they didn't know mine. Most didn't wave as they drove down the street, and some frightened me (the drug dealers in the rental house across from me). I rarely spoke with anyone on my street except Wilda, the widow next door. I had more in common with her than with my friends from college or my sisters back east, who were getting married and having babies. (My sister, Susan, and my friend, Kathy, who'd traveled in Europe with me, had both married the Steves they'd been dating on that trip.)

Believing there was a blueprint for constructing a life, I sought this knowledge. I signed up for a workshop called, "Focus on Being Single." I wanted to discover how people fashioned lives, how one found pleasure in the company of one's self. I was the only attendee in my twenties; the rest were divorced men and women in their thirties and forties, each offering ways to meet suitable mates, ski trips, supermarkets, even church, which I found depressing. This was not the empowering seminar I'd hoped for, and afterward when a man wearing a large key chain attached to his belt loop indelicately asked for my phone number in the parking lot, I felt more flawed and aberrant than when I'd woken up that morning.

After Sally moved back east, I stayed home alone every Saturday night, renting movies, drinking beer, waltzing around my very own living room in my very own mortgaged home, burdened with ankle weights, listening to Patsy Cline singing, *I go walking, after midnight, searching for you.* I couldn't seem to make friends or find the life I was sure existed out in the world, a dazzling, glamorous adult life: attending soirees, wearing chic ensembles, sipping cocktails, swirling ice cubes.

I kept trying. I signed up for jitterbug lessons, something I'd always wanted to learn. At the first lesson, I met my partner, Duane, a fortyish man who reeked of the fruity fragrance of pipe tobacco, and who used a product to slick his hair. I instantly despised Duane for who he was *not*: the handsome, suave dance partner of my dreams. One night each week I had to hold Duane's leathery hands. Our palms were sweaty in each other's clasp, which felt too intimate. I had to touch his shoulder, allow his fingertips on the small of my back.

All the other couples in the class were actual couples, who'd signed up together. Why had I thought jitterbug lessons would be teeming with lively single people? The jitterbug is a dance for two, a dance that both partners must know with exactitude, must be in sync to perform. Still, I couldn't quit as I yearned to because I'd feel guilty leaving Duane in the lurch, partnerless, abandoned on the dance floor. His loneliness was burdensome, reminding me of my own. And so each week I attended the class and each week I grew increasingly frustrated with Duane for he could not keep a beat and had no rhythm.

Duane sensed that my frustration was not just with his dance steps, but with him. We quietly seethed as we smiled and stepped along. We tried the Cinnamon Roll. Duane whipped me back toward him, yanking my shoulder so that the bone in my arm seemed to momentarily float loose in the socket. Instead of curling in toward Duane as a Cinnamon Roll spirals toward its center, I resisted and crashed into his chest. I wallowed in self-pity. Why was my life filled with error and fluke and oddity? What type of bad karma surrounded me? I imagined a tiny dark nimbus hovering above my head, the opposite of the steaming, protective Cream of Wheat bowl in the television ad I remembered from childhood.

Duane and I grew contemptuous of each other. Clearly I was not the partner Duane imagined either. When he threw my body out for a spin, it was too hard, as if he wanted to throw me away. When he stepped on my foot, I hissed, "*Left* foot, Duane." Duane and I did not dance together; we sparred. I began to hate myself, the self I was in his presence, this angry rigid self.

One night after a lesson, toward the end of the ten-week course, Duane invited me for a beer at a local blues and jazz club, and I accepted. I liked the idea of going to a club on a week night, which seemed cosmopolitan, cityish, sophisticated, part of a life, part of living, even if I had Duane as the envoy into this exotic, interesting life. The club was impressively divey, and the blues singer was excellent, up from Detroit where the real blues lived.

We sat at a sticky table, drank a beer, talked above the music. I realized that Duane was a nice man, decent, even interesting since he knew a great deal about jazz. He was suffering from his recent divorce. I told him about Steve. Something came unknotted then and we relaxed. We even enjoyed the remaining few lessons.

I've danced the jitterbug only once since that class, with my father at his second wedding, two years after Steve died. My father was a graceful dancer, a strong lead. I was tipsy and reckless, and many times aloft as he twirled me around the dance floor. I spent myself dancing that day, pure embodied joy. I could probably perform a Cinnamon Roll today, though I've forgotten the more intricate moves of the jitterbug, only the basics: join, separate, rejoin. But beyond foot placements, beyond spins and lifts, there was something else I took from those lessons that has stayed with me: give yourself over to the spirit of the dance, to the choreography of each day, whatever its rhythm. Lead with your heart.

Coda

Once when I was flying back to Michigan after visiting my family in Massachusetts, as I reached for my packet of pretzels, the flight attendant grabbed my left hand. "Oh, your ring is beautiful. Are you engaged?"

"Yes," I said. It was easier than explaining.

I was relieved that she didn't pursue the subject, ask when I was to be married. I would have had to answer *never* because Steve was dead.

Since he'd given me the ring for my birthday in June, two months before he died, I'd worn the diamond faithfully on the fourth finger of my left hand, which was why the flight attendant assumed that I was engaged. The weight of the ring on my finger was reassuring and it felt right, like the cloak of grief that shrouded me, that I couldn't shake off. Sometimes the ring felt like a badge I'd earned for love, like a girl scout merit award for loyalty.

One day, though, about a year after Steve died, I took the ring off to wash dishes and set it on the kitchen windowsill. After drying my hands, I picked up the ring, but something stopped me from slipping it back on my finger. There was nothing different about that day, though I had recently turned twenty-eight. Time was moving forward, but I was still hitched to a past, with no promise of a return to it, or of a future. Wearing that diamond, I was forever engaged, in nuptial limbo, a phantom relationship: the heart goes on loving long after its object is gone. I was betrothed but never to wed. The origin of the word betrothed is *truth*, but the ring was a lie. I could not *engage* with Steve for the simple reason that he was not alive.

At first I felt guilty tucking the ring in my jewelry box, wedged in a fold of red velvet, especially as I saw the diamond every day when I dressed for work. But over time it was liberating, my hands free and unencumbered with the heaviness of the ring and all it symbolized. Near the end of his life, Steve would say he wanted me to find someone else to love; I always answered that I didn't want anyone else. After he died, I believed wholly that I'd never again fall in love again. I couldn't imagine it, couldn't envision it. But three years later, to my surprise, I did fall in love, and after that relationship ended, I fell in love again, and then again.

It strikes me now how strange it was that I went around wearing an engagement ring from a dead man. But I remember how hard it was to accept that Steve was gone. In the final weeks of his life, he was in so much pain that he could bear only light kisses, so in bed each night we held hands like two shy teenagers. With my hand clutching his as we fell asleep, I'd half-convinced myself that when his soul slipped away, I'd be carried along with him. After he died, I was momentarily surprised to find myself still alive.

Now, decades later, I still have the ring. Every once in a while, when I open my lockbox to store documents, I see the ring in its small black box, in a baggie with the certificate from LeRoy's Jewelers, guaranteeing that the diamond was cut and polished "by a master craftsman" who created a "gem of complete beauty." The diamond sparkles brilliantly and the gold band still shines, unsullied by everyday wear.

When Steve gave me the ring, I was underweight from the stress of caring for him and the sadness of witnessing him suffer, so I had a sizer attached to it. Now the ring no longer fits; it's too small, and that seems apt. My experience of caring for Steve is indelible, etched in my heart, so I don't need the ring to *always remember and never forget*. I take comfort, though, knowing that the ring is there in my fireproof lockbox, safe in my safe.

Acknowledgments

In a memoir, one must select memories and events to include, and others to omit. There was much happening in the lives of Steve's family and mine during the time he was ill, but these stories are not mine to tell; including them would have made them seem merely incidental as my focus of this memoir was Steve's and my experience of love, illness, and loss.

I am indebted to many people who helped make this book possible, especially Allen Gee, Stephen Kiernan, and the late Donald Jordan and the Jordan family, who make possible the Donald L. Jordan Prize for Literary Excellence. I'm grateful to Peter Selgin for the gorgeous cover, to Gwen Grafft for formatting, and everyone at Columbus State University Press. Thanks also to Bethany Snead, Candice Lawrence and the team at the University of Georgia Press.

I'm grateful to Lisa Taddeo, who selected my essay, "The Murmur of Everything Moving," as the winner of the *Sewanee Review* contest in 2023, and to the editors of the SR for publishing it.

Many people read work-in-progress and shared their wisdom and time. For this generosity, I thank: Brenda Brueggemann, Stephanie Grant, Michelle Herman, E.J. Levy, Sandra Miller, Nancy Sferra, and Melanie Rae Thon. Special thanks to Andre Dubus III for his kind and generous support.

I am grateful to the Medical Records Department of the City of Hope Cancer Center in Zion, Illinois (formerly American International Hospital), whose employees copied, gratis, over 1,000 pages of medical records for me. I'm most grateful for Dr. Ranulfo Sanchez, Steve's primary oncologist, and to all the physicians, nurses, technicians and other staff in 1986 and 1987 who offered Steve excellent and compassionate care. To Dr. Cendra Lynn in Ann Arbor, a truly gifted counselor—after all these years, thank you for saving me from despair; I'm grateful for your intuitive powers, your generosity, your sage counsel.

252 | ACKNOWLEDGMENTS

I received financial help for this book from The Ohio State University, the MacDowell Colony, the Maine Arts Commission, Change, Inc., and the University of Massachusetts Lowell. To these institutions, their founders and their keepers, I am indebted.

Thanks to Steve's parents, Bill and Louise, who gave me Steve. I'm grateful for their faith during his illness (when I had none); in the end, their faith gave Steve comfort. I'm grateful to Steve's family for their help and support during his illness, and to me after his death. Thank you to Steve's children, who brought joy to my life.

Thank you to my Ann Arbor friends and coworkers, who were so kind to me. Vickie Norfleet asked to "borrow my laundry," a small but generous gesture to ease my burden. Heartfelt thanks to Marga and Stephen Hampel, who never gave up on me when I withdrew after Steve passed, never answering the phone, hiding in my grief. They invited me into their home, fed me delicious dinners, and brought me back into the world of the living with their love and friendship.

I owe so much to my siblings, Susan Watson, Sally Stanton, Joanne King, Patrick Stanton, Barbara Goodhue, Michael Stanton, Colin Stanton, who've always been supportive of my writing. Thanks especially to Sally, my only sibling in Michigan during this time, who returned me to myself in those years, and to art and joy and humor. Thanks, especially, to my mother, whose advice to "follow my heart" has been my lifelong lodestar.

About the Author

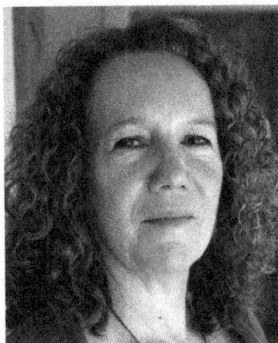

Maureen Stanton is the author of *Body Leaping Backward: Memoir of a Delinquent Girlhood*, winner of the Maine Literary Award for memoir and a *People Magazine* "Best Books Pick"; and *Killer Stuff and Tons of Money: An Insider's Look at the World of Flea Markets, Antiques, and Collecting*, winner of the Massachusetts Book Award in nonfiction and a *Parade Magazine* "12 Great Summer Books" selection. Her essays have received the *Iowa Review* prize, the *Sewanee Review* prize, Pushcart Prizes, the *American Literary Review* award, and the Thomas J. Hruska award from *Passages North*. She's been awarded fellowships from the National Endowment for the Arts, the Maine Arts Commission, the MacDowell Colony, and the Virginia Center for Creative Arts. She teaches creative writing at the University of Massachusetts Lowell.

The Donald L. Jordan Endowment was established in 2016, in part, to facilitate the formation of Columbus State University Press, which was officially formed in 2021. CSU Press is pleased to recognize Mr. Jordan as the founder of the press, which serves as the publishing venue for the Donald L. Jordan Prize for Literary Excellence, and for The Nature Series at DLJ Books. DLJ Books has been installed as a permanent imprint at the press. Mr. Jordan's foresight made CSU Press a reality, and we are grateful for his generosity. Mr. Jordan passed away on May 15, 2023 after a very successful business career. The author of literary novels, short stories, and works of non-fiction, he was also particularly interested in helping other writers attain publication.